Questions and Answers Set:

Book 1
2018 Edition

By Stu Silverstein, M.D., FAAP

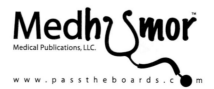

MedHumor Medical Publications, Stamford, Connecticut

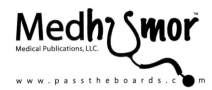

www.passtheboards.com

Published by:
Medhumor Medical Publications, LLC
1127 High Ridge Road, Suite 332
Stamford, CT 06905 U.S.A.

All rights reserved. No part of this book may be reproduced, or transmitted in any form or by any means, electronic or mechanical, including photocopying, recording or by any information storage and retrieval system without written permission from the author, except for the inclusion of brief quotations in a review.
One-panel cartoons are copyright ©·2000-2018 Medhumor Medical Publications, LLC.

Copyright © 2000, 2008, 2016, 2018 Medhumor Medical Publications, LLC

ISBN: **978-0-692-05862-6**

First Edition Copyright © 2000 Medhumor Medical Publications, LLC
Second Edition Copyright © 2008 Medhumor Medical Publications, LLC
Third Edition Copyright © 2016 Medhumor Medical Publications, LLC
2018 Edition Copyright © 2018 Medhumor Medical Publications, LLC

Printed in the United States of America

This book is designed to provide information and guidance in regard to the subject matter covered.
It is to be used as a study guide for physicians preparing for the General Pediatric Certifying Exam administered by the American Board of Pediatrics. It is not meant to be a clinical manual. The reader is advised to consult textbooks and other reference manuals in making clinical decisions. It is not the purpose of this book to reprint all the information that is otherwise available, but rather to assist the Board Candidate in organizing the material to facilitate study and recall on the exam. The reader is encouraged to read other sources of material, in particular picture atlases that are available.

Although every precaution has been taken in the preparation of this book, the publisher, author, and members of the editorial board assume no responsibility for errors, omissions or typographical mistakes. Neither is any liability assumed for damages resulting from the direct and indirect use of the information contained herein. The book contains information that is up-to-date only up to the printing date. Due to the very nature of the medical profession, there will be points out-of-date as soon as the book rolls off the press. The purpose of this book is to educate and entertain.

**If you do not wish to be bound by the above,
you may return this book to the publisher for a full refund.**

Publisher:	MedHumor Medical Publications, LLC Stamford, CT
VP/Content Development:	Stuart Silverstein, MD, FAAP Clinical Director Firefly After Hours Pediatrics, LLC Stamford, CT Assistant Clinical Professor Emergency Medicine New York Medical College
Senior Editor:	Lourdes Geise, MD, FAAP
Vice President/ Operations:	Brian Cahn 3rd Year Medical Student Albert Einstein College of Medicine
Design/Copy Editor:	Antoinette D'Amore, A.D. Design addesign@videotron.ca
Cover Designers:	Rachel Mindrup www.rmindrup.com Leo Rosas Vickers www.leorosasvickers.com

About the Author

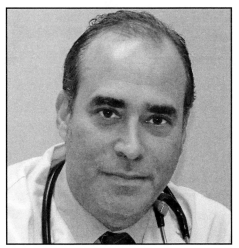

Dr. Stu Silverstein is the founder and CEO of Medhumor Medical Publications, LLC which began with the publication of the critically acclaimed "Laughing your way to Passing the Pediatric Boards"™ back in the spring of 2000. Word spread quickly that finally there was a book out there that turned a traditionally daunting process into one that was actually fun and enjoyable. This groundbreaking study guide truly "Took the Boredom out of Board review"® with reports from our readers that they were able to reduce their study and review time in half. Those who were taking the exam for the 2nd time not only passed but increased their scores dramatically.

Their supplementary pediatric titles have also been crtically acclaimed. Medhumor Publications LLC, has since expanded their catalogue to include a title for the USMLE Step 3 Neurology Board exams, and Neonatology exams.

The concept of the "Laughing your way to Passing the Boards"™ and Medhumor Medical Publications, LLC were conceived by Dr. Silverstein. He brought his years of experience in the field of Standup Comedy and Comedy writing after he realized the critical need for a study guide that spoke the language of colleagues rather than the language of dusty textbooks. His work as a Standup Comedian and Medical Humorist has frequently been featured in several newspapers, radio programs and TV shows, including the New York Times, WCBS newsradio in NY City, as well as World News Tonight with Peter Jennings.

Dr. Silverstein has also served as a contributing editor for the Resident and Staff Physician annual board review issue and has authored numerous articles on medical humor. He has served on the faculty of the Osler Institute Board Review course, UCLA Pediatric Board Review course and several local board review courses. He is the co-author of "What about Me? Growing up with a Developmentally Disabled Sibling" written with Dr. Bryna Siegel, professor of Child Psychiatry, the University of California San Francisco. Dr. Silverstein is in demand as a lecturer for residency programs on successful preparation for the pediatric board exam.

In addition to writing, lecturing, and expanding the scope of Medhumor Medical Publications, LLC., Dr. Silverstein is the Clinical Director for Firefly After Hours Pediatrics, a subacute emergency practice. Dr. Silverstein is an Assistant Clinical Professor of Emergency Medicine at the New York Medical College in Valhalla, New York.

Question and Answers Set: Book 1 2018 Edition

In putting together the 2018 edition of our Question and Answer series we did our utmost to incorporate the suggestions of our readers who successfully passed the General Pediatric Board Exam as well as the Recertification Exam.

Each book now contains more than 400 questions each broken down by subspecialty. This allows the reader to focus on areas that need improvement.

All questions have been reviewed and revised based on the content specifications published by the American Board of Pediatrics. The infectious disease and preventive medicine questions were updated based on the most up to date information published in the online edition of the AAP "Red Book".

We hope that these updated *Question and Answer* books will continue to serve those for whom passing the pediatric certification and recertification exams is the next ticket to be punched.

—Stuart Silverstein, MD, FAAP
Stamford, CT

Table of Contents

Questions 1

- Nutrition 3
- Preventive Pediatrics 7
- Poisons and Toxins 11
- Fetus and Newborn 13
- Fluids and Lytes 20
- Genetics 23
- Allergy and Immunology 28
- Infectious Disease 30
- Inborn Errors of Metabolism 39
- Endocrinology 42
- GI 49
- Pulmonary 54
- Cardiology 58
- Heme onc 62
- Renal 69
- Genitourinary 73
- Neurology 76
- Musculoskeletal 83
- Dermatology 88
- Rheumatology 92
- Ophthalmology 96
- ENT 98
- Adolescent Medicine and Gynecology 106
- Sports Medicine 110
- Substance Abuse 112
- Disorders of Cognition, Language and Learning 114
- Behavior and Mental Health 115
- Psychosocial 117

Critical Care	122
Emergency Medicine	124
Pharmacology and Pain Management	132
Research and Statistics	134
Ethics for Primary Care Physicians	136
Patient Safety and Quality Improvement	138

Answers 141

Nutrition	143
Preventive Pediatrics	146
Poisons and Toxins	149
Fetus and Newborn	151
Fluids and Lytes	158
Genetics	160
Allergy and Immunology	163
Infectious Disease	165
Inborn Errors of Metabolism	172
Endocrinology	175
GI	180
Pulmonary	185
Cardiology	188
Heme onc	191
Renal	197
Genitourinary	200
Neurology	202
Musculoskeletal	207
Dermatology	211
Rheumatology	215
Ophthalmology	218
ENT	220
Adolescent Medicine and Gynecology	227
Sports Medicine	230

Substance Abuse	232
Disorders of Cognition, Language and Learning	234
Behavior and Mental Health	235
Psychosocial	237
Critical Care	241
Emergency Medicine	242
Pharmacology and Pain Management	247
Research and Statistics	248
Ethics for Primary Care Physicians	251
Patient Safety and Quality Improvement	253

References 255

Questions

Nutrition

1) Breast milk is known to contain each of the following *EXCEPT*:

   A) IgA
   B) Immunomodulating agents
   C) IgG
   D) Anti-inflammatory agents
   E) Anti-microbial agents

2) Match each numbered description on the left to a vitamin deficiency on the right

   1) Leading cause of blindness worldwide
   2) Hemolytic anemia
   3) Hemorrhagic disease of the newborn
   4) Peripheral paralysis and muscle weakness
   5) Stomatitis and seborrheic dermatitis

   (A) Phylloquinone
   (B) Retinol
   (C) Riboflavin
   (D) Thiamine
   (E) Tocopherol

3) Match each numbered item on the left to its corresponding toxicity on the right.

   1) Liver toxicity
   2) Vasodilator
   3) Nephrocalcinosis

   (A) Ascorbic acid
   (B) Niacin
   (C) Tocopherol

4) Calciferol deficiency can result in each of the following *EXCEPT*:

   A) High serum phosphatase levels
   B) Infantile tetany
   C) Poor growth
   D) Pharyngeal ulcers
   E) Osteomalacia

5) **Niacin deficiency results in each of the following *EXCEPT*:**

   A) GI distress
   B) Xerophthalmia
   C) Dementia
   D) Skin manifestations
   E) Pellagra

6) **You are evaluating a 9 month infant who has been increasingly fussy over the past 2 days. The family has recently returned from a trip abroad where the only available formula was evaporated milk which the child was fed exclusively on the trip. You note that the child seems reluctant to being touched and has some peripheral edema and swelling of the gums.**

   X-ray findings include ground glass appearance of the bones, thinning of the cortices, and calcified cartilage at the metaphysis.

   The most appropriate treatment at this time would be:

   A) Removal of the child from the home.
   B) Iron supplementation
   C) Calcium and vitamin D supplementation
   D) Ascorbic acid supplementation
   E) Fortified infant formula

7) **You are evaluating a 4 year old boy presenting with increasing irritability and headache over the past 3 days despite ibuprofen. Additional findings include some joint aches and lethargy. The child has not been experiencing nausea or vomiting and has remained afebrile. Lumbar puncture reveals an elevated opening pressure with no red or white blood cells.**

   The most likely explanation for the physical findings would be:

   A) Aseptic meningitis
   B) Trauma
   C) Retinol deficiency
   D) Retinol toxicity
   E) Migraine headaches

Questions

8) You are evaluating a dark skinned 12 month baby boy who as been exclusively breast fed up until now. The boy was born at 31 weeks gestation and was in the NICU for 1 week receiving supplemental oxygen for 3 days.

On physical exam, the baby is below the 10th percentile for weight and height. You note some bowing of the legs and increased width of the wrists. Laboratory findings are significant for decreased serum calcium and phosphate with an elevated alkaline phosphatase level.

These findings are best accounted for by:

A) Vitamin D deficiency
B) Vitamin E deficiency
C) Vitamin A deficiency
D) Iron deficiency anemia
E) Cystic fibrosis

9) Which of the following would be the most appropriate treatment of a child with mild dehydration who is tolerating clear fluids without emesis?

A) IV fluids and hospital admission
B) IV fluids, oral rehydration and discharge home on clear liquids for 24 hours
C) Clear liquids for 24 hours and then advance to a diet of bananas, rice, apples, toast, and tea
D) Oral rehydration and discharge home on diet of bananas, rice, apples, toast and tea
E) Oral rehydration and discharge on his regular diet as tolerated

10) You have admitted a 13 year old boy because of complications related Crohn's disease. You need to decide whether to provide nutrition with enteric formula via an NG tube or parenteral nutrition. The most important factor in making your decision would be:

A) The presence or absence of an anal fistula
B) The degree of inflammation noted on colonoscopy
C) The presence or absence of fever
D) The results of plain abdominal film
E) The presence or absence of digestive enzymes

11) Which of the following is true regarding home prepared versus commercial baby food products in infants?

A) Home prepared foods decreased the risk for development of food related allergies.
B) Honey can be added provided it has been properly stored
C) Home prepared products must be used immediately, discarding any unused portions
D) Pureed home prepared foods can be frozen and used later
E) Home prepared vegetables offer no advantage over bottled vegetables

12) Each of the following are associated with breastfeeding except:

A) Reduced maternal risk for type 2 diabetes
B) Reduced risk for postpartum depression
C) Reduced risk for breast cancer
D) Reduced weight loss in the immediate postpartum period
E) Reduced risk for ovarian cancer

Preventive Pediatrics

13) Which of the following statements is true with regards to cholesterol levels in children?

   A) Screening for hypercholesterolemia should be started at age 1
   B) In the absence of a positive family history for hypercholesteremia, screening will pick up an insignificant number of cases
   C) An elevated HDL cholesterol level is a worrisome finding in children
   D) Children older than 2-1/2 years of age should receive no more than 35% of their caloric intake from fat
   E) Hypercholesteremia in children is due exclusively to diet and genetic predisposition.

14) Hyperlipidemia can be found in each of the following conditions EXCEPT:

   A) Sideroblastic anemia
   B) Hyperthyroidism
   C) Renal disease
   D) Cushing syndrome
   E) Hypothyroidism

15) Intake of each of the following is associated with hyperlipidemia EXCEPT:

   A) Isotretinoin
   B) Ethanol
   C) Methanol
   D) Oral contraceptives
   E) Steroid supplements

16) Which of the following is true regarding a 12 year old with a previous history of pertussis?

   A) A previous diagnosis of pertussis is easy to confirm
   B) DTaP vaccine is contraindicated with a previous history of pertussis disease
   C) Tdap vaccine is contraindicated with a previous history of pertussis disease
   D) Tdap should be administered according to routine recommendations.
   E) The duration protection after B pertussis infection is lifelong and no further immunization is indicated

17) An 8-year-old boy cut his foot on a rusty nail in the family garage. He received DTaP immunization at 2, 4, and 15 months. Which of the following is the most appropriate to give today?

   A) Td
   B) Tdap
   C) DTP
   D) DTaP
   E) DT

18) The parents of a healthy 1-month-old infant are concerned that he has colic because he is crying a lot. They note that his 4-year-old sibling had colic and that his father is "climbing the home entertainment center in frustration." Which of the following statements is TRUE regarding crying in infants?

   A) As long as the infant-crying to father-whining ratio is less than 1:2 it is normal
   B) Parental fear or anxiety plays a role in colic
   C) Crying associated with flexion of the arms and legs is diagnostic of colic
   D) Infants tend to cry more during the first month after birth
   E) Newborn infants cry only in response to hunger

Questions

19) Of the following, the most significant problem associated with fatal accidents and injuries in adolescents is:

   A) Depression
   B) Ethanol consumption
   C) Poor education on safety issues
   D) Parental permissiveness
   E) Dropping out of high school

20) In which of the following clinical situations is the MMR vaccine contraindicated?

   A) A child with ALL in remission who has not received chemotherapy for 5 months
   B) A child with ITP who is receiving IV IG
   C) A child with sickle cell disease
   D) A child with stable HIV infection
   E) A child with OM

21) Each of the following would be considered a contraindication for participation in contact sports *EXCEPT*:

   A) Splenomegaly
   B) Hepatomegaly
   C) Acute diarrhea with dehydration
   D) Impetigo
   E) Single testicle

22) Regarding suicide among adolescents, each of the following statements is true *EXCEPT*:

   A) Suicide attempts are more frequent among females
   B) The number of suicides completed is higher among males
   C) Suicide is the most common cause of death among adolescents
   D) Only a fraction of adolescent suicide attempts come to medical attention
   E) Firearms are the most prevalent method used in completed suicides

23) Which of the following would correlate best with *chronic alcohol abuse*?

   A) Elevated serum gamma glutamyl transferase
   B) Hypoglycemia
   C) Metabolic acidosis
   D) Decreased mean corpuscle volume
   E) Elevated blood alcohol levels

24) Each of the following is true regarding drug abuse among adolescents *EXCEPT*:

   A) Weapon carrying is associated with alcohol use
   B) Fighting is more commonly seen with adolescents who use anabolic steroids
   C) Teens who use anabolic steroids are at higher risk to abuse other drugs
   D) Violent behavior is more common among adolescents who use drugs
   E) Violent behavior is more common among male drug users than female drug users

25) Which of the following are the 2 most effective tools in preventing tooth decay in the general population?

   A) Fluoride varnish application/Oral Fluoride Supplements
   B) Community fluoridation /fluoride mouth rinse
   C) Community fluoridation/fluoride toothpaste
   D) Fluoride Chewing gum/ Fluoride Varnish Application
   E) Community Fluoridation/ Oral Fluoride Supplements

26) You are evaluating an infant with difficulty swallowing and poor tone. Each of the following would be appropriate in distinguishing transient neonatal myasthenia gravis from infantile botulism *EXCEPT*:

   A) Edrophonium testing
   B) Age of onset
   C) Maternal history
   D) Presence of constipation
   E) Poor long term prognosis with infantile botulism

Poisons and Toxins

27) You are evaluating an 8 year old boy who drank from a bottle left on the kitchen counter that he thought was water, after he drank a " few swigs " he spit it out because it tasted horribly. Since drinking this stuff, he has been going through some coughing fits and is complaining of being very tired. On examination his respiratory rate is 65 and there you note crackles and fine expiratory wheezing on examination. Which of the following would the most appropriate first step in managing this patient?

   A) Inactivated charcoal
   B) Albuterol/Oxygen supplementation
   C) Intravenous ethyl alcohol
   D) Budesonide/Oxygen supplementation
   E) Upper endoscopy

28) Which of the following is true regarding lead toxicity in children?

   A) Calcium, iron and vitamin C enhance lead absorption
   B) Behavioral concerns are rarely due to lead exposure
   C) Blood lead levels as low as 5 micrograms/ dL warrant evaluation for diet and environmental exposure
   D) Chelation therapy can reverse the neurocognitive effects of lead toxicity
   E) Annual universal screening of all children is mandatory

29) Ingestion of each of the following medications can lead to hypotension with the exception of:

   A) Clonidine
   B) Lorazepam
   C) Iron
   D) Amphetamine
   E) Imipramine

30) Each of the following is associated with amphetamine toxicity *EXCEPT*:

   A) Vomiting
   B) Mydriasis
   C) Increased muscle strength
   D) Fever
   E) Hyperreflexia

31) Each of the following is consistent with salicylate toxicity *EXCEPT*:

   A) Dehydration
   B) Hyperthermia
   C) Hypoglycemia
   D) Hyperkalemia
   E) Hypoxia

Questions

Fetus and Newborn

32) A full term, small-for-gestational-age baby is born to a 25 year old G3 P1 Mom. There was no prolonged rupture of membranes (PROM) and the mom is group B strep negative. She has received good prenatal care. The baby was born 4 hours ago and is being breast-fed, yet remains somewhat irritable, jittery and tachypneic. Since it is 3 in the morning, you are also irritable and jittery so you stop by the vending machine to pick up a couple of Kit Kats® to tide you over. You arrive and find a well-appearing infant with a normal exam and bilateral 5-10 beat ankle clonus. The first thing you should do at this point is:

   A) Order a head ultrasound because, given the neurological findings, CNS asphyxia is very likely
   B) Order a full sepsis workup and start ampicillin and gentamicin without delay
   C) Quit your job immediately (the hours and the Kit Kats® are horrible) and sign a non-compete 30-year agreement with this infant as your agent, because clearly he has rhythm and is the next "Counting Crows" Ben Ulrich
   D) Check the serum glucose and get ready for a D10 W bolus
   E) Get some more Kit Kats® and microwave granola bars; it's gonna be a long night and morning

33) The most appropriate antibiotic regimen for empiric treatment of neonatal sepsis in the NICU setting is:

   A) Ampicillin
   B) Gentamicin
   C) Cefotaxime
   D) Ampicillin and gentamicin
   E) Ampicillin and cefotaxime

34) An infant with cystic fibrosis is being supplemented with medium chain triglycerides (MCT). When, on rounds, you are asked why, you correctly answer:

   A) Chain rhymes with sane and gets things through
   B) MCT is partially water-soluble and can be directly transported into the portal vein
   C) Micelle formation is facilitated by MCT
   D) Absorption in the distal small bowel is facilitated
   E) Because of its stimulatory effect on bile acid production and secretion

35) A newborn is cyanotic with each feeding. The cyanosis resolves as soon as the feeding stops. You strongly suspect choanal atresia and order the following to make a definitive diagnosis:

A) Skull films
B) Head CT
C) Attempt to pass an NG and confirm position with chest film
D) A feeding of pureed sea conch imported from the Cayman Islands; looked good on the "Learning Channel"
E) Head ultrasound

36) A 2-week old infant has become increasingly irritable and been feeding poorly. He has a maculopapular rash on his trunk as well as hepatosplenomegaly. An ophthalmological exam reveals some inflammation of the retina. Head CT reveals some calcifications. The MOST LIKELY diagnosis is:

A) Toxoplasmosis
B) Congenital CMV
C) Congenital syphilis
D) Herpes simplex
E) Child Abuse

37) The diagnosis above is best made via:

A) Head CT
B) Serum IgM
C) Serial serology measurement
D) Urine culture
E) Brain biopsy and EEG

38) Match each infant reflex to the age on the right when it disappears in healthy full term infants:

1) Palmar grasp   (A) 2 months
2) Plantar grasp   (B) 4 months
3) Automatic stepping   (C) 6 months
4) Moro reflex   (D) 9 months
5) Money grasp   (E) Law school grad

39) A full-term child is born to a 28-year-old mother with moderately controlled diabetes. Each of the following is a complication seen in infants of diabetic mothers *EXCEPT*:

A) Hypertension
B) Congenital anomalies
C) Persistent pulmonary hypertension
D) Polycythemia
E) Hypercalcemia

40) A 32-hour-old baby with Apgars of 9/9 who had been feeding well and appeared healthy until now, has developed intermittent episodes of cyanosis. The oxygen saturations are in the high 50s with no improvement with oxygen supplementation. The infant does not appear to be in respiratory distress. The most appropriate NEXT step would be:

A) Start IV antibiotics
B) Endotracheal intubation
C) Give a 20cc/ kg IV NS bolus
D) Start IV prostaglandins
E) Start IV indomethacin

41) An otherwise healthy full term newborn develops bilious vomiting at 24 hours of age. The MOST appropriate next step in managing this patient would be:

A) Abdominal ultrasound
B) Rectal stimulation to induce a bowel movement
C) Rectal exam and stool guaiac
D) NG tube, NPO, and 24-hour observation
E) Abdominal x-ray

42) An 18-month-old toddler who is being evaluated for the first time since birth has global developmental delay, and microcephaly. Essential testing at this time would include each of the following *EXCEPT*:

A) Screening for congenital syphilis
B) Head CT
C) Full developmental assessment
D) Evaluation for vision and hearing
E) TORCH titers

43) Of the following, the neonate at greatest risk of developing infection with hepatitis B is a neonate whose mother:

A) Received immune globulin
B) Was treated for preeclampsia
C) Recently had a blood transfusion
D) Is a recent immigrant from Lichtenstein
E) Is a drug user

44) A healthy infant is born by forceps delivery in the breech position. At 9 days of age, she is brought for evaluation because of skin lesions. Mother's prenatal history is negative. Which of the following findings is *most likely* to require immediate hospitalization?

A) Flat bluish discoloration over the posterior spine and buttocks
B) Scattered vesicles with erythematous bases confined to the buttocks
C) Pustular melanosis
D) Hard nodules with erythematous overlying skin confined to the lateral buttocks
E) Pigmented macules

Questions

45) You are evaluating a 3-hour-old infant who is the product of an uncomplicated full term gestation vaginal delivery. The respiratory rate is 43 with no respiratory distress. The hands and feet are noted to be cyanotic; otherwise the physical examination is within normal limits. The *most* appropriate next step in managing this infant would be:

   A) Obtain a CXR
   B) Measure the arterial blood gas
   C) Request a cardiology consultation
   D) Administer oxygen via nasal canula
   E) Place the infant under a radiant warmer

46) Which of the following BEST explains what is measured by a prenatal non-stress test?

   A) Evaluates how much stress the average neonatal fellow can endure during the month of July
   B) Evaluates the response of the infant's HR to drug induced uterine contractions
   C) Evaluates fetal lung maturity
   D) Evaluates the fetal autonomic nervous system integrity
   E) Evaluates the volume of amniotic fluid present

47) You are evaluating a 3 day old infant who presents with abdominal distension without emesis. A KUB reveals large dilated loops of bowel with no air noted in the rectosigmoid area. On physical examination the anus is patent.

   The most appropriate study in this scenario is:

   A) Upper GI series
   B) Endoscopy
   C) Contrast enema
   D) Abdominal ultrasound
   E) Abdominal CT

Copyright 2018 by Medhumor Medical Publications, LLC

48) A one month old male infant is brought in by a frantic father because of enlargement of both breasts[1] and some milky white discharge.

Prominent breast buds are noted with no inflammation or erythema. You note bilateral descended testicles and normal genitalia. Which of the following is the most appropriate next step?

A) IV antibiotics
B) Head CT
C) Reassurance
D) Review father's medication and diet
E) Review mother's medications and diet

49) You are evaluating a 5-week-old infant who appears well but has lost weight since birth. You obtain the following lab values:

Sodium of 135, potassium of 3.2, chloride of 102, and serum bicarb of 8. Arterial blood gas reveals a pH of 7.22 and a PCO2 of 28. The *most likely* diagnosis would be:

A) Pulmonary disease
B) Distal renal tubular acidosis
C) Proximal renal tubular acidosis
D) Polycystic kidney disease
E) Maple syrup urine disease

50) A full-term infant is born via spontaneous vaginal delivery. Very thick particulate meconium is noted. The delivery was precipitous, leaving no time for the gynecologist to do DeLee suctioning on the perineum. You are attending the delivery as the pediatrician.[2] The baby is crying vigorously and has a one-minute Apgar of 8. Which of the following would be the MOST appropriate management in this situation?

A) Since the one-minute Apgar is 8, endotracheal intubation is not necessary
B) Since the one-minute Apgar is not 8, direct visualization via neither laryngoscopy nor endotracheal intubation is necessary
C) Direct visualization via laryngoscopy is indicated
D) Endotracheal intubation and suctioning to remove meconium are indicated
E) Due to the clinical status, no intervention is indicated

---

1 In the baby not the father.
2 As opposed to the videographer.

51) A very frantic nurse and mother call you to the nursery. A one-day-old infant has a rash that is concentrated on the trunk. The rash started out as papules but is now yellow, with pustules surrounded by red skin. The infant is clinically doing well. Maternal history is unremarkable. Upon further evaluation you would likely find:

A) A high WBC on CBC left shift and bacteremia
B) A high WBC on CBC predominately eosinophils
C) Wright stain of the lesion with primarily neutrophils
D) Wright stain of the lesion with primarily eosinophils
E) Tzanck smear with intranuclear inclusions

52) During prenatal screening, an elevated alpha-fetoprotein level is noted. Each of the following are legitimate concerns *EXCEPT*:

A) Twins
B) Omphalocele
C) Open spina bifida
D) Trisomy 21
E) Congenital nephrotic syndrome

53) Each of the following is associated with dietary protein intolerance in children *EXCEPT*:

A) IgE mediated food hypersensitivity
B) Typically involves, egg, soy and milk proteins
C) Vomiting and diarrhea
D) Heme positive stools
E) Failure to thrive

54) Hypochloremic, hypokalemic metabolic alkalosis would be seen in:

A) Congenital adrenal hyperplasia
B) Pyloric stenosis
C) Protein intolerance
D) Cystic fibrosis
E) Distal renal tubular acidosis

Fluids and Lytes

55) Please match the diagnoses on the left with the lab values on the right:

			Na	K	Cl	Glucose	BUN	Urine Sp.Gr.Dx
1)	Lab error	(A)	152	4.3	118	95	28	1.002
2)	Pseudohyponatremia	(B)	152	4.2	119	73	22	1.020
3)	Hyponatremic dehydration	(C)	122	4.0	90	76	4	1.029
4)	SIADH	(D)	121	4.2	84	80	20	1.021
5)	Hypernatremic dehydration	(E)	122	4.2	107	450	10	1.017
6)	Diabetes insipidus	(F)	119	4.3	105	80	10	1.011

56) A 20-month-old infant who has congenital heart disease is currently receiving digoxin and furosemide. Which of the following sets of drug-related conditions are most likely to develop in this patient?

A) Hyponatremia and hyperkalemia
B) Hypernatremia and hyperkalemia
C) Hyperchloremia and hypokalemia
D) Hypernatremia and hypokalemia
E) Hypochloremia and hypokalemia

57) Which of the following is best represented by an arterial pH of 7.35, PCO_2 of 30 mm Hg, PO_2 of 110 mm Hg, and a serum bicarbonate concentration of 18 mEq/L?

A) Respiratory acidosis with metabolic compensation
B) Respiratory alkalosis with metabolic compensation
C) Metabolic alkalosis with respiratory compensation
D) Metabolic acidosis with respiratory compensation
E) Lab error

58) A 6-month-old infant has a 5-day history of producing 13 to 14 mostly watery stools a day. He has a blood pressure of 55/35 mm Hg, a heart rate of 170, a RR of 55, and is afebrile. The peripheral pulses are palpable but weak and his skin is cold and mottled. The patient is producing urine. After successfully starting an IV, your NEXT step would be to:

A) Congratulate yourself for starting an IV on such a "difficult stick"
B) Administer D_5 0.45% Normal Saline 10 cc/kg over 20 minutes
C) Administer Ringers lactate 20 cc/kg over 20 minutes
D) Administer D_5 0.2% Normal Saline 20cc/kg over 10 minutes
E) Administer oral rehydration

59) A 2% concentration of glucose (111 mmol/L) in solution for oral rehydration is chosen because at this concentration:

A) Coupling of intestinal sodium transport is optimal
B) Secretory diarrhea is prevented
C) Hypoglycemia is prevented
D) Hepatic glycogen stores are adequately replaced
E) Insulin secretion is appropriately reduced

60) Each of the following is a cause of metabolic alkalosis *EXCEPT*:

A) Laxative abuse
B) Organophosphate poisoning
C) Diuretic therapy
D) Pyloric stenosis
E) Bartter syndrome

61) Each of the following is an adverse consequences of severe alkalemia *EXCEPT*:

A) Arteriole constriction
B) Reduction in coronary blood flow
C) Hypoventilation
D) Hypocapnia
E) Hypokalemia

62) You are evaluating a 7 week old male with increasing severity of projectile vomiting.

Lab studies include:

Sodium – 130
Potassium – 3.5
Chloride – 90
Bicarb 35

Which of the following is likely to reveal the underlying disorder?

A) Plain x-ray
B) 17 hydroxy (OH) progesterone level
C) Abdominal ultrasound
D) pH probe study
E) Air contrast enema

63) Which of the following is characteristic of heat stress?

A) Decreased exercise performance
B) Confusion
C) Nausea and vomiting
D) Core temperature between 100.4 F and 104 F
E) Core temperature greater than 104 F

Genetics

64) Each of the following is associated with a delayed eruption of teeth *EXCEPT*:

A) Gardner's syndrome
B) Hypothyroidism
C) Hypopituitarism
D) Ectodermal hypoplasia
E) NHL hockey syndrome

65) Each of the following symptoms is associated with Treacher Collins syndrome *EXCEPT*:

A) Small jaw
B) Intellectual disability
C) Ear abnormalities
D) Lower eyelid abnormalities
E) Conductive hearing loss

66) Each of the following is inherited in an autosomal dominant inheritance pattern *EXCEPT*:

A) Waardenburg syndrome
B) Aicardi syndrome
C) Retinoblastoma
D) Tuberous sclerosis
E) Achondroplasia

67) Edwards Syndrome (Trisomy 18) is associated with all of the following *EXCEPT*:

A) Hypoplastic nails
B) Rocker bottom feet
C) Bicornate uterus
D) Punched-out scalp lesions
E) Horseshoe kidney

68) A couple in your practice is expecting their first child. Mom has myotonic muscular dystrophy and they would like to know the odds of this child having the disorder. You tell them:

   A) 50% if the child is male and 0% if the child is female
   B) 25%
   C) 50%
   D) 100%
   E) It is the same as the general population

69) Patau syndrome (Trisomy 13) is associated with each of the following *EXCEPT*:

   A) Scalp defects
   B) Congenital heart defects
   C) Rocker bottom feet
   D) Microphthalmia
   E) Holoprosencephaly

70) The chances of an asymptomatic girl, whose brother has cystic fibrosis (C.F.), being a carrier of C.F. is closest to:

   A) 0%
   B) 33%
   C) 25%
   D) 66%
   E) 100%

71) You have attended a routine C-section and suspect the baby has Down's syndrome. Each of the following will increase your index of suspicion for Down's syndrome *EXCEPT*:

   A) Cleft palate
   B) Wide gap between first and second toe
   C) Duodenal atresia
   D) Redundant skin, posterior neck
   E) Single transverse palmar crease

Questions

72) It is December 26th and you have 40 patients in your waiting room not counting the ones you are actually evaluating in your examination rooms. You get an e-mail from the Department of Public Health. One of the patients in your practice has been identified as "positive PKU" (phenylketonuria). In addition to diet counseling and placing this infant on Lofenalac®, you need to order the following:

A) A Thriller Vanilla Lofenalac® cocktail for yourself tonight (Lofenalac® and vanilla Absolute® vodka)
B) Serum NH_4 every 6 months
C) Anion gap and B12 levels
D) Homocysteine levels
E) Testing for tetrahydrobiopterin deficiency

73) The parents of one of your patients would like to know the odds of their having a child with hemophilia A. The father has a brother with the disorder but he himself is unaffected.

A) 0%
B) 25%
C) 50%
D) 100%
E) 125%

74) The pattern of inheritance of myoclonic epilepsy is BEST described as:

A) Occurring through patrilineal inheritance
B) Occurring through matrilineal inheritance
C) X-linked inheritance patterns
D) Due to abnormalities in mitochondrial DNA
E) B and D

75) A 9 year old boy is well known to your practice because he is very friendly whenever he comes to the office and speaks a lot, although content is lacking. His physical exam is most notable for small hands, feet, and genitalia. He was noted to be floppy as an infant.

Genetic studies would reveal:

A) Trisomy 13
B) Deletion on chromosome 13
C) Deletion on chromosome 15 inherited from his father
D) Deletion on chromosome 15 inherited from his mother
E) You identify this as Bill Clinton, pass GO and collect $200

76) Which of the following BEST describes the inheritance pattern of tuberous sclerosis?

A) X-linked recessive
B) X-linked dominant
C) Autosomal dominant
D) Autosomal recessive
E) Random mutation

77) In the following set of questions, decide if each numbered choice applies to (A) only, (B) only, both (C), or neither (D):

1) Pulmonic stenosis
2) Coarctation of the aorta
3) Webbed neck
4) Chromosomal abnormality
5) Can affect females

(A) Turner's syndrome
(B) Noonan syndrome
(C) Both
(D) Neither

78) You are at a cocktail party enjoying the appetizers and decent California white wine with an excellent bouquet. The word is out that you are a doctor and some investment banker with a lot less personality than the wine's bouquet pulls you aside and says, "Doc, I have a question. My sister is going to marry a guy whose brother has cystic fibrosis. She doesn't have it. What are the chances of their having a kid with cystic fibrosis?" Your answer is:

A) 1 in 4
B) 1 in 20
C) 1 in 150
D) 1 in 200
E) How the heck do I know? I am not a geneticist, now how about some stock tips you creepy loser?

Allergy and Immunology

79) A patient with a C6 complement deficiency of C6 would be MOST at risk for infection with which of the following?

   A) *Staphylococci*
   B) Candida
   C) Retroviruses
   D) Mycobacteria
   E) *Neisseria*

80) A 2-year-old boy with eczema has had recurrent respiratory infections including *Pneumocystis carinii* pneumonia. Lab studies show thrombocytopenia and normal serum immunoglobulin concentrations. Which of the following is the most likely diagnosis?

   A) Chronic disease
   B) AIDS
   C) DiGeorge syndrome
   D) Thrombotic thrombocytopenia
   E) Wiskott-Aldrich syndrome

81) Each of the following is true regarding ataxia telangiectasia EXCEPT:

   A) It is an autosomal dominant condition
   B) Presents with regression of motor milestones
   C) Is associated with recurrent sinopulmonary infections
   D) Findings often include depressed IgA levels
   E) It has an increased risk of malignancy

82) Each of the following is true regarding chronic granulomatous disease *EXCEPT:*

    A) Most forms are inherited in an X-linked recessive pattern
    B) It can be diagnosed with the *Nitroblue tetrazolium test (NBT)*
    C) Bowel obstruction is a possible complication
    D) Prophylactic treatment with trimethoprim/sulfamethoxazole and/or itraconazole is indicated
    E) This is a defect of chemotaxis

83) Immediate treatment of acute anaphylactic reactions includes

    A) Oral diphenhydramine
    B) Oral corticosteroids
    C) 0.01 mg/kg of epinephrine (1:10,000) SQ
    D) 0.01 mg/kg of epinephrine (1:1000) SQ
    E) 0.1 mg/kg of epinephrine (1:1000) SQ

84) Which of the following is the most common trigger of life threatening anaphylaxis in children?

    A) Snake bite
    B) Bee sting
    C) Food
    D) MMR vaccine
    E) Penicillin

Infectious Disease

85) You are treating a child with amoxicillin for Lyme disease documented on serology. The child now presents with a high fever with chills. Mom reports to your office as a drop-in appointment to find out "why you are not treating this correctly". You tell her:

   A) She is correct. You are treating "Lime" disease not "Lyme" disease; without a medical spell checker you are lost!
   B) You will switch the child's medication to doxycycline, the optimal choice.
   C) You will administer a shot of IM ceftriaxone and increase the dosage of amoxicillin
   D) This is consistent with treatment
   E) Her child must be allergic to amoxicillin.

86) Which of the following drugs used in the treatment of tuberculosis is associated with optic neuritis?

   A) Ethambutol
   B) Pyrazinamide
   C) Rifampin
   D) Isoniazid
   E) Streptomycin

87) A 5-year-old girl presents with two red papules on her right arm, a temperature of 38.5C that started yesterday, a poor appetite, and a headache. Prominent lymph nodes are noted in the right axilla along with a maculopapular rash on her trunk and conjunctivitis of the left eye. History is noncontributory. The *most likely* diagnosis is:

   A) Rocky Mountain spotted fever
   B) Kawasaki disease
   C) Rubeola
   D) Bartonella henselae infection
   E) Pasteurella multocida infection

88) A 9-month-old infant has had a fever with a T max of 39.2C along with bloody diarrhea that lasted for 2-3 days. The infant is now afebrile. Stool cultures taken at the time of illness are now positive for *Salmonella* species. A blood culture taken at the same time is negative. Which of the following would be MOST appropriate?

   A) Amoxicillin
   B) Trimethoprim /sulfamethoxazole therapy
   C) Ceftriaxone
   D) Erythromycin
   E) Observation

89) A 12-year-old girl has been exposed to a classmate at school who was diagnosed with *Streptococcal* pharyngitis by throat culture. Which of the following is the MOST appropriate recommendation to the parents?

   A) The girl should be removed from school for one week
   B) The girl should be treated with penicillin and return to school 24 hours after starting treatment
   C) Throat cultures should be obtained from all children in the class, treatment pending culture results
   D) The girl should be brought in for evaluation only if symptoms of a *Streptococcal* infection appear
   E) The girl should receive IM Bicillin®

90) Each of the following is true regarding infantile botulism *EXCEPT*:

   A) Constipation is a late finding
   B) Gentamicin should never be used.
   C) Botulism toxin blocks the release acetylcholine from the presynaptic neuron
   D) Botulism toxin is the active ingredient of Botox® injections
   E) Treatment is largely supportive.

91) A child with which of the following would appropriately be excused from attending their first-grade class tomorrow after you made the diagnosis tonight??

   A) Ear infection
   B) EBV infection
   C) Tinea corporis
   D) *Strep* throat
   E) Asymptomatic *Salmonella* colonization

92) After visiting his uncle last month, a 7 year-old boy presents with fever, muscle aches, and a headache. On exam, you note severe conjunctivitis and preauricular lymphadenopathy. Serological testing confirms infection with Francisella tularensis. Which of the following antibiotics could be used to treat this boy?

   A) Vancomycin
   B) Tetracycline
   C) Doxycycline
   D) Ciprofloxacin
   E) Gentamicin

93) It is 4 AM and you are covering the pediatric ER, and you just "cleared the waiting room". Your next patient is well known to you since it is a 4-year-old who has chronic paronychia infections. The most likely cause of this chronic infection is:

   A) The desire of this family to make sure you do not sleep while on call
   B) *Pseudomonas aeruginosa*
   C) *Staph aureus*
   D) *Candida albicans*
   E) Group A beta-hemolytic Strep

Questions

94) A boy in your practice is being treated for meningococcemia. In addition to appropriate antibiotic treatment, which of the following additional measures would be the MOST appropriate?

   A) Immunization of contacts with meningococcal vaccine
   B) Oral administration of rifampin to family members
   C) Oral administration of sulfadiazine to family members
   D) Assessment of splenic function in the patient during convalescence
   E) Assessment of adrenal function in the patient during convalescence

95) A 3-year-old child presents with rhinorrhea, fever, conjunctivitis, and pharyngitis. What is the MOST likely causative agent?

   A) Adenovirus
   B) Beta-hemolytic Strep
   C) Epstein-Barr virus
   D) *Staph aureus*
   E) *Haemophilus influenzae* type b

96) An 18-month-old has a one-week history of cough, tachypnea, and diminished appetite, and now presents with a 2-day history of high fever. On physical exam, the child is grunting and retracting with some abdominal distension. CXR shows a right middle lobe infiltrate with a large pleural effusion. Which of the following organisms is the MOST likely culprit here?

   A) Mycoplasma pneumoniae
   B) *Chlamydia pneumoniae* (TWAR)
   C) Adenovirus
   D) Staph aureus
   E) *Moraxella Catarrhalis*

97) A 15-month-old child presents with a generalized rash for 3 days with a temperature of 38.1°C. On physical exam, you note generalized tender erythematous skin with denuding of the skin over parts of the trunk, with the base of each of these areas appearing to be clear and shiny. You also notice flaccid bullae with crusting around the mouth and nose. Physical findings are otherwise normal. Which of the following is the most likely diagnosis?

A) Erythema multiforme major
B) Staphylococcal scalded skin syndrome
C) Epidermolysis bullosa
D) Bullous impetigo
E) Kawasaki syndrome

98) You are called upon to take care of a 4-year-old boy who is HIV positive. He presents with weight loss, malaise, abdominal pain, and diarrhea. By isolating which of the following pathogens would you be MOST justified in diagnosing AIDS?

A) *Salmonella* species
B) *Mycobacterium avium* complex
C) *Campylobacter* species
D) Streptococcus pneumoniae
E) Haemophilus influenzae

99) A 12-year-old boy presents with a 1-day history of pain in his right thigh. On physical exam, his temperature is 39.3C with a HR of 110 and RR of 34. Pain is noted with palpation of the distal portion of his affected thigh and on movement of the right knee. However, there is no swelling or effusion noted on his knee. His CBC is remarkable for a WBC of 17,500 mm3 with a left shift. ESR is 51. Which organism is the MOST likely guilty party?

A) *H flu* type b
B) Group B beta-hemolytic Strep
C) Staphylococcus aureus
D) *Salmonella* species
E) Gnu painus

100) Following treatment for H. pylori gastritis, which of the following would be valid tests to document the eradication of the pathogen?

   A) Fecal H. pylori antigen
   B) Endoscopy with biopsy
   C) Urease breath test
   D) H. pylori IgG
   E) A,B,C

101) You are caring for a child who attends day care with a child who is in the pediatric intensive care unit for meningococcal sepsis. The child and the family left on vacation 5 days ago, which was the last day the child was in the same classroom with the index case.

   The story has made national news and the parents saw it on CNN and are calling you for advice. Your advice to them is:

   A) Seek medical attention if the child develops fever or a rash
   B) The child and parents need chemoprophylaxis
   C) The child needs chemoprophylaxis
   D) Stop watching CNN and start watching the Daily Report with Jon Stewart.
   E) Since the child was exposed 5 days ago no intervention is needed

102) You are evaluating a 7 year old child who presents with a papular rash along with several vesicular lesions that started on the trunk and now has spread to his face and extremities. One day prior to the development of the rash, he developed a fever of 102.3. His immunization status is unknown.

   He appears well but cannot return to school without a definitive documented diagnosis. Which of the following tests would help establish the correct diagnosis in the shortest period of time?

   A) Viral culture
   B) Molecular amplification
   C) Skin biopsy
   D) Direct fluorescent antibody
   E) Polymerase chain reaction

103) You are treating a 12 year old with a community acquired skin infection which has not responded to treatment with cephalexin. You suspect the infection is due to a methicillin resistant Staph aureus infection. Which one of the following antibiotics would be most appropriate for this patient?

A) Amoxicillin/clavulanic acid
B) Cefdinir
C) Doxycycline
D) Levofloxacin
E) Amoxicillin

104) Which one of the following is the most appropriate *rapid* test for influenza virus?

A) Direct fluorescent antibody
B) Enzyme immunoassay antigen detection
C) Viral culture
D) Serum IgM titers
E) Polymerase chain reaction

105) Which of the following antibiotics would be least effective in treating Listeria monocytogenes?

A) Chloramphenicol
B) Penicillin
C) Trimethoprim-sulfamethoxazole
D) Cefotaxime
E) Gentamicin

106) Each of the following would be appropriate steps for a CMV seronegative pregnant mother to take regarding the care of her 2 year old child *EXCEPT*:

A) Sleeping in the same bed should be completely eliminated
B) No kissing on or near the child's mouth
C) No changing of diapers or handling the child's laundry
D) Assume that any child younger than 3 years of age is secreting CMV in their saliva and urine
E) No sharing towels or washcloths with the child

107) Which one of the following would be most appropriate routine confirmation of cat scratch disease in a child?

A) Lyme node biopsy and culture
B) Wound culture
C) Antigen skin testing
D) Enzyme immunoassay (EIA)
E) Polymerase chain reaction

108) Which of the following is true regarding rabies in humans?

A) Prior rabies immunization provides protection against CNS disease
B) The diagnostic test of choice is direct fluorescent antibody staining
C) The diagnostic test of choice is reverse transcriptase-polymerase chain reaction
D) More than 50% of cases may have no documented history of exposure
E) The presence of high CSF rabies titers confirms previous disease

109) Which of the following would be the most appropriate treatment of a child bittern by a bat that was not isolated?

A) Reverse transcriptase-polymerase chain reaction testing
B) Wash the wound and treat with cephalexin only
C) Infiltrate the wound with rabies immunoglobulin
D) Provide HDCV today and on days 3,7,14, and 28
E) C and D

110) You are presented with a patient whose HBsAb is positive. The HBsAg and HBcAb are negative. What is the correct interpretation of these results?

A) I am sorry I have to read the question again
B) Chronic hepatitis B infection
C) Active hepatitis B infection
D) Immune after recovery from hepatitis B infection
E) Immune following hepatitis B vaccine

111) Which of the following is true regarding Herpes simplex virus (HSV) infection

   A) HSV virus is transmitted through breast milk
   B) Neonatal infection is associated with fetal and maternal antibodies against HSV
   C) Congenital infection is associated with fetal and maternal antibodies against HSV
   D) Treatment for neonatal HSV infection should not be started viral culture confirmation
   E) Lower rates of transmission are associated with maternal seronegativity

112) You are evaluating a 13-year-old girl who presents with increasing fatigue for the past 10 days. She developed a sore throat 5 days ago and has had a fever of 101-102 F for the past 2 days. She was seen at a drive by telemedicine center at a rest stop while on vacation and started on amoxicillin-clavulanate for presumed strep pharyngitis. She has not gotten any better. In fact, she is having difficulty swallowing. You note on exam that her pharynx is scarlet red with white exudate and the tonsils are enlarged and almost touching. She has large tender bilateral cervical lymph nodes. In addition, you note abdominal tenderness with her spleen palpable 2 cm below the costal margin. You also noted a flat macular papular red rash that is irregularly spaced with raised borders. Her routine immunizations are up to date.

   Which of the following would be the most likely diagnosis:

   A) Strep pharyngitis
   B) Scarlet fever
   C) Systemic allergic reaction
   D) Infectious mononucleosis / amoxicillin rash
   E) Acute Epiglottitis

Inborn Errors of Metabolism

113) In the following set of questions, for each numbered word or phrase, choose the lettered heading that is MOST CLOSELY ASSOCIATED with it. Lettered headings may be selected once, more than once, or not at all.

1) "Mousy odor" urine
2) "Sweaty socks odor" urine
3) Hypertonic and tachypneic during first week of life
4) "Dark urine"

(A) Isovaleric acidemia
(B) Alcaptonuria
(C) Maple syrup urine disease (MSUD)
(D) PKU

114) In the following set of questions, decide if each numbered choice applies to (A) only, (B) only, both (C), or neither (D):

1) Elevated serum ceruloplasmin
2) Elevated serum copper levels
3) Acute hepatic failure
4) Treated with IM penicillin
5) Elevated tissue copper levels
6) X-linked

(A) Wilson's disease
(B) Menkes Kinky Hair Syndrome
(C) Both
(D) Neither

115) A 3 week-old exclusively breast-fed infant presents with a one week history of jaundice and vomiting, one day of fever and irritability, a bulging fontanelle, and hepatomegaly. Which of the following is the most likely diagnosis?

A) Fructose aldolase deficiency
B) Fructose-1, 6 biphosphate deficiency
C) Glycogen storage disease type 1
D) Neonatal adrenoleukodystrophy
E) Galactosemia

116) A child born with which of the following disorders is at GREATEST risk for experiencing a cerebral vascular accident?

A) Maple syrup urine disease
B) Pompe disease
C) Pompous disease
D) Homocystinuria
E) Hunter syndrome

117) You are evaluating a 5-month-old infant for poor weight gain and intermittent vomiting of several weeks' duration. Three weeks ago the infant was weaned from breast milk and started on cow milk, baby food vegetables, and fruits.

On physical examination you note that the infant is irritable, and jaundiced, with a liver palpable 3-4 cm below the right costal margin. Which of the following is the *most likely* diagnosis?

A) Hypothyroidism
B) Galactosemia
C) Hereditary fructose intolerance
D) Sensitivity to beta lactoglobulin
E) Glycogen storage disease type 1

118) You are evaluating a boy with swelling of his left knee although he has not sustained any trauma. He has not been outdoors much, is afebrile, and also is complaining of red eyes with no discharge. The rest of the physical exam is benign.

On further investigation, which of the following would you also expect to find?

A) Kayser Fleisher rings
B) Malar rash
C) Dysuria
D) Evidence of physical abuse
E) Evidence of self mutilation

Questions

119) Soy formula would be most appropriate in a child with which of the following conditions?

A) Maple syrup urine disease
B) Pompe disease
C) Allergic colitis
D) Cow milk allergy
E) Galactosemia

120) You are evaluating an 18 month old boy whose growth and development are blunted. He is hypotonic with hepatosplenomegaly. You note a retinal cherry red spot on funduscopic exam.

The most likely diagnosis is:

A) Tay Sachs disease
B) Niemann Pick disease
C) Wolman disease
D) Wilson disease
E) Autism

Endocrinology

121) Each of the following is more commonly associated with diabetes mellitus type 2 than type 1 **EXCEPT**:

   A) Obesity
   B) Insulin resistance
   C) Earlier age of onset
   D) treatment with metformin
   E) Acanthosis nigricans

122) Which of the following can be used to definitively distinguish diabetes mellitus type 1 from type 2?

   A) Family history of type 2 diabetes
   B) Serum C- Peptide level
   C) Acanthosis nigricans
   D) Ketoacidosis
   E) Beta cell autoantibody level

123) You are evaluating a 16 year old boy who is obese, with dark velvety skin on his neck and chest and a family history of type 2 diabetes. His fasting glucose is 110 mg/dL and 2 hour glucose challenge test is 230 mg/dL. Which of the following is true regarding this patient?

   A) He meets the American Diabetes Association criteria for diabetes mellitus
   B) He should be admitted for IV insulin
   C) He should be started on a trial of glyburide
   D) He should start treatment only if he is symptomatic
   E) He does not meet the diagnostic criteria for diabetes

124) In normal female pubertal development, which of the following represents the normal sequence?

   A) Full Pubarche → Full thelarche → menarche
   B) Partial Pubarche → Partial menarche → thelarche
   C) Menarche → thelarche → Welder's arc
   D) Full Thelarche → Full pubarche → menarche
   E) Partial Thelarche → Partial pubarche → menarche

125) During which Genital SMR stage does the growth spurt occur on average in boys?

   A) SMR 1
   B) SMR 2
   C) SMR 3
   D) SMR 4
   E) SMR 5

126) During which Breast SMR stage does the growth spurt occur on average in girls?

   A) SMR 1
   B) SMR 2
   C) SMR 3
   D) SMR 4
   E) SMR 5

127) Your patient is a 12 year old boy who, according to his family and teachers, has become increasingly more emotional and hyperactive and has not been able to sleep well at all. The symptoms have developed gradually over the past year and a half. You work in a small rural town that is not even recognized by your car's GPS. The nearest community hospital is roughly twice the size of your dashboard GPS.

Despite a perfectly normal physical exam, you suspect the patient is hyperthyroid. Which of the following is true regarding patients who are hyperthyroid?

A) They may occasionally be jaundiced
B) The absence of exophthalmia rules out Graves disease
C) Hepatomegaly is a common finding
D) Pretibial myxedema is a common finding
E) All of them have will have elevated TSH levels

128) **The first sign of pubertal development in males is:**

A) Axillary hair
B) Facial hair
C) Testicular enlargement
D) Peak growth velocity
E) Unwillingness to separate from his Cleveland Brown football helmet in mixed company

129) **The first sign of pubertal development in females is:**

A) Axillary hair
B) Pubarche
C) Hiding the Cleveland Brown helmet from their male counterparts
D) Thelarche
E) Menarche

130) In the following set of questions regarding short stature, decide if each numbered choice applies to (A) only, (B) only, both (C), or neither (D):

1) Delayed bone age
2) Normal adult height
3) Family history
4) Precocious puberty
5) Checked for in neonatal screening

(A) Hypothyroidism
(B) Constitutional growth delay
(C) Both
(D) Neither

131) For each number, choose the letter on the graph that best corresponds.

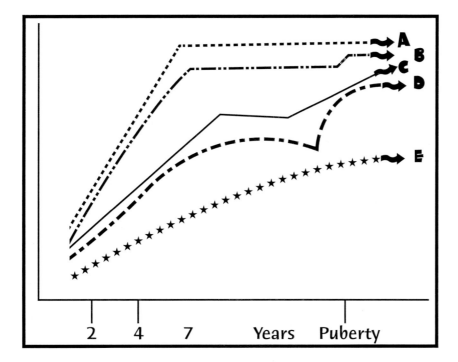

For the following questions, select the line on the graph that best corresponds to the correct diagnosis for short stature.

1) Craniopharyngioma
2) Hypothyroidism
3) Untreated congenital adrenal hyperplasia
4) Constitutional delay
5) Genetic short stature

132) You are presented with a 14-year-old girl whose height and sexual maturation differ from those of her peers. On physical examination, her height is lower than the 5%ile, and weight is in the 10%ile. Temperature is 37.1 C, HR is 72/minute, RR is 18, and BP is 95/67 in the arms and 105/86 in the legs. You note a broad chest, scattered pigmented nevi, and hyperconvex fingernails and toenails. Tanner is stage 1 for breast development and stage 2 for pubic hair.

Each of the following is likely to be associated findings EXCEPT:

A) 45, X Karyotype
B) Horseshoe kidney on renal ultrasound
C) 45, XXY Karyotype
D) Bicuspid aortic valve on cardiac echo
E) Pedal edema

133) A 15-year-old underwent an uneventful surgical resection of a suprasellar tumor. His hospital course was unremarkable. Ten days later he is experiencing lethargy coupled with dizziness. On physical examination his skin turgor is poor, eyes appear sunken, and he has orthostatic hypotension. Serum glucose concentration is 42 mg/dL. Serum sodium concentration is 124 mEq/L and serum potassium concentration is 6.1 mEq/L. Based on these findings, the MOST likely diagnosis is:

A) SIADH
B) Septic shock
C) Adrenal insufficiency
D) Cushing syndrome
E) Diabetes insipidus

134) Each of the following is a common complication of prednisone therapy EXCEPT:

A) Memory loss
B) Glucose intolerance
C) Growth retardation
D) Cosmetic effects
E) Increased risk for infection

Questions

135) The parents of a 10-year-old boy are concerned about their son's short stature. Height and weight are around the 5%ile for age, and his growth velocity is 5 cm/year. The father is 160 cm tall, and the mother is 147 cm tall. Of the following, the MOST likely cause of this patient's short stature is:

   A) Congenital adrenal hyperplasia
   B) Hypothyroidism
   C) Familial short stature
   D) Growth hormone deficiency
   E) Constitutional growth delay

136) You are asked by a boy's parents to estimate their son's adult height. Assuming that both parents have reached their genetic potential, you tell them that the BEST estimate can be determined by:

   A) Pulling a random number out of both parents' hats and dividing by 3
   B) The mean parental height
   C) The mean parental height plus 6.5 cm
   D) The mean parental height minus 6.5 cm
   E) The son's height will most likely mirror dad's height

137) A 16-year-old girl is concerned about her obesity. Menarche occurred at 12 years of age and her menstrual periods have been irregular. Her cognitive development has been normal and she has been otherwise healthy. Her height is at the 85%ile and weight >95%ile. She has moderate papulonodular acne and abundant facial hair. Which of the following is the MOST likely diagnosis?

   A) Hypothyroidism
   B) Prader-Willi syndrome
   C) Anabolic steroid abuse
   D) Stein-Leventhal syndrome
   E) Gonadal dysgenesis

138) On physical exam you note what you believe to be a thyroid nodule. Which of the following would be a reassuring factor that the nodule is benign?

   A) Older than 15
   B) Nodule larger than 2 cm
   C) Nodule smaller than 2 cm
   D) Younger than 15
   E) Adjacent cervical lymphadenopathy

139) Which of the following is true regarding the diagnosis and treatment of thyroid malignancies in children?

   A) The diagnostic yield of fine needle biopsy is independent of the skill of the physician taking the sample and the pathologist doing the reading
   B) The diagnostic yield is independent of the size of the nodule
   C) Follicular adenomas can be distinguished by fine needle biopsy alone
   D) Fine needle biopsy is the gold standard for preoperative diagnosis of thyroid nodules
   E) Hemorrhage and abscess formation are common after fine needle abscess formation

GI

140) You are evaluating a 3 year old child with a history of failure to thrive and frequent loose stools. Giardia has been ruled out. Your presumptive diagnosis is gluten-sensitive enteropathy. The definitive test to diagnose gluten-sensitive enteropathy is:

   A) Have the child attend the annual Gluten and Garlic festival and watch the results from the reviewing stand
   B) The gluten challenge test
   C) A serum antigliadin antibody measurement
   D) A small bowel biopsy
   E) Stool gluten degradation test

141) Which of the following is consistent with a diagnosis of chronic non-specific diarrhea in the toddler?

   A) Flatulence that has guests leaving on schedule.
   B) Normal growth
   C) Bloody stools
   D) Severe abdominal pain
   E) Vomiting

142) You are asked to be one of the keynote speakers at the "Passing the boards without passing a stool" conference. The title of your lecture is "Chronic Diarrhea, Will It Get you in the End?" After describing the stool velocity and splatter patterns, you describe the hallmarks of the stool found in chronic non-specific diarrhea in the toddler. Your list, consistent with a diagnosis of chronic non-specific diarrhea in the toddler, is correct with the _EXCEPTION_ of:

   A) Stool pH less than 5 and positive reducing substances
   B) Occult blood
   C) Rarely passing stools during sleep
   D) Mostly occurring in the morning
   E) Watery diarrhea

143) Match the GI condition on the left with the clinical description on the right.

1) Fecal impaction
2) Partial small bowel obstruction
3) Crohn's disease
4) Mesenteric venous obstruction

(A) Bloody diarrhea followed by seizure
(B) Malodorous green stools with fever
(C) Left lower quadrant fullness
(D) Pressure tenderness on the right lower quadrant along with fever and joint aches
(E) Teen using oral contraceptives
(F) Vomiting, weight loss and anorexia

144) In the following set of questions, decide if each numbered choice applies to (A) only, (B) only, both (C), or neither (D):

1) Skipped lesions are common
2) Associated with ankylosing spondylitis
3) Surgery is curative

(A) Crohn's disease
(B) Ulcerative colitis
(C) Both
(D) Neither

145) A 5-month-old infant presents with poor weight gain and a voracious appetite. The parents note that the child has foul smelling greasy stools that "require a gas mask", according to the parents.[3] On physical examination you note a rather small, thin infant that also appears to be pale. You politely confirm the parents' assessment of the stool as you discretely dispose of it through a trap door you create *with your bare hands* on the spot.

You obtain a CBC, which reveals a low white blood cell count and a low hematocrit. You obtain two negative sweat chloride tests. Incidental x-ray finding reveals metaphyseal dysostosis. Which of the following is the MOST likely diagnosis?

A) Cystic fibrosis
B) Diamond-Blackfan syndrome
C) Inflammatory bowel disease
D) Metaphyseal dysplasia
E) Shwachman-Diamond syndrome

---

[3] Foul-smelling stools are often described, yet isn't this redundant? Are there any other kinds of stools?

146) Which of the following approach is MOST appropriate with uncomplicated gastroesophageal (GE) reflux?

A) Barium swallow
B) PH probe sleep study
C) 24-hour apnea monitoring at home
D) Pulmonary consultation
E) Observation over time

147) The MOST common symptom of gastroesophageal (GE) reflux in infants is:

A) Projectile vomiting
B) Passive regurgitation
C) Apnea
D) Poor weight gain
E) Aspiration pneumonia

148) Which of the following is BEST associated with tocopherol deficiency?

A) Megaloblastic anemia
B) Photophobia and blurred vision
C) Glossitis
D) Hemolytic anemia
E) Poor wound healing

149) Anorexia, slowed growth, drying and cracking of the skin, hepatosplenomegaly, and increased intracranial pressure would MOST likely be the result of an EXCESS of:

A) Niacin
B) Ascorbic acid
C) Riboflavin
D) Cyanocobalamin
E) Retinol

150) Deficiency of cyanocobalamin can be associated with each of the following conditions *EXCEPT*:

   A) Homocystinuria
   B) Juvenile pernicious anemia
   C) Celiac disease
   D) Methylmalonic aciduria
   E) Dermatitis

151) Match the numbered causes of infantile vomiting with the lettered descriptions on the right.

   1) GER (gastroesophageal reflux)
   2) Rumination
   3) Necrotizing enterocolitis
   4) Duodenal atresia

   (A) Does not occur during sleep
   (B) Polyhydramnios
   (C) Normal phenomenon in nearly all infants
   (D) 10% to 35% of the affected infants are full term

152) Match the numbered cause of vomiting with the lettered description on the right.

   1) CNS etiology
   2) Gastroesophageal reflux
   3) Rumination
   4) Gastrointestinal cow milk allergy
   5) Allergic gastroenteropathy

   (A) Rapid drop in hematocrit
   (B) Associated with weight loss, hypoalbuminemia, and diarrhea
   (C) May present with chronic respiratory problems and rhinitis
   (D) Can occur with posturing
   (E) May respond to behavioral interventions

153) Each of the following is true regarding Wilson disease *EXCEPT*:

   A) It is inherited in an autosomal dominant fashion
   B) It may present with a mixed conjugated and unconjugated hyperbilirubinemia
   C) It is rarely manifests before age 3
   D) Copper chelation is one form of treatment
   E) Zinc acetate, which prevents absorption of copper from the GI tract, is another form of treatment

Questions

154) Each of the following are possible complications of GERD in infants *EXCEPT*:

   A) Feeding refusal
   B) Poor weight gain
   C) Apnea
   D) Anemia
   E) Upper airway symptoms

155) Each of the following statements regarding Rotavirus is true *EXCEPT*:

   A) The primary mode of transmission is fomite
   B) It is mostly seen during the winter
   C) Rotavirus has been isolated from the respiratory tract
   D) Delayed gastric emptying plays no role in vomiting seen during acute infection
   E) Adults are more likely to be asymptomatic

156) Each of the following is true regarding abdominal migraines *EXCEPT*:

   A) It is more common in males
   B) It can present as episodic epigastric pain
   C) It can present as episodic periumbilical pain
   D) Family history is often present
   E) Acute episodes can last an hour or more

157) Which of the following is true regarding acute pancreatitis in children?

   A) Epigastric pain in the absence of pain radiating to the back is rarely due to pancreatitis
   B) Amylase and lipase levels twice normal levels is consistent with a diagnosis of acute pancreatitis
   C) Normal pancreas on abdominal ultrasound rules out pancreatitis
   D) Amylase and lipase levels 3 times normal levels is consistent with a diagnosis of acute pancreatitis
   E) The incidence of pancreatitis in children is much lower than adult populations

Pulmonary

158) Coughs, coughs, coughs—we see them all the time. Which one of the following statements regarding coughs in children is TRUE?

   A) Coughs from an upper respiratory infection are most prominent during the day
   B) Coughs due to pneumonia are most prominent at night, during naps, and the early morning.
   C) The older a child is, the more likely a persistent cough is due to pneumonia.
   D) Grunting is a common finding in infants with pneumonia
   E) A persistent cough is a common presentation of pneumonia in the newborn period

159) A previously healthy 18-month-old boy presents with sudden onset of cough for 2 days. The cough began while he was in the living room watching "The Wiggles". He is afebrile with no sick contacts. Wheezing is heard over the right lower lobe. Of the following, the *most likely* diagnosis is:

   A) An appropriate response to watching grown men prancing around pretending to be kids.
   B) GE reflux
   C) Asthma
   D) Cystic fibrosis
   E) Foreign body aspiration

160) A 14-year-old intermittent asthmatic in your practice wants to play basketball and exercise is one of his triggers. Which of the following statements is the best advice to offer this family?

   A) The boy should not participate in a strenuous sports program
   B) Inhaled steroids should be administered prior to and after exercise
   C) He should be started on daily montelukast
   D) Oxygen should be available on site
   E) Beta-agonist bronchodilators should be administered 30 minutes prior to strenuous exercise

161) A 6-month-old infant is status post TE fistula repair and presents with wheezing and expiratory stridor. The MOST likely explanation would be:

A) Recurrence of TE fistula
B) Laryngomalacia
C) RSV bronchiolitis
D) Tracheomalacia
E) Lobar pneumonia

162) Each of the following is a risk factor for asthma persisting after adolescence EXCEPT:

A) Family history of asthma
B) Recurrent viral illnesses
C) Elevated IgE levels
D) Eosinophilia
E) Seasonal allergies

163) A 15-year-old boy with cystic fibrosis presents with rapid onset of severe respiratory distress and chest discomfort. He has been fully compliant with his daily regimen of antibiotics and other care. The symptoms can be best explained by:

A) Pseudomonas pneumonitis
B) Acute bronchospasm
C) Acute pneumothorax
D) Septic pleural effusion
E) Acute pulmonary insufficiency

164) A 10-year-old girl has had a cough for the past 2 months. Findings on physical examination are normal except for a harsh, loud cough. Results of a CBC are normal. A CXR and sinus x-rays are normal. Peak expiratory flow rates are normal before and after exercise. A tic disorder is suspected of being the underlying cause. Which of the following would best support the tentative diagnosis?

A) Control of cough with albuterol therapy
B) A family history of a tic disorder
C) Persistence of cough after administration of codeine
D) Absence of cough during sleep
E) A positive response to phenothiazine therapy

165) A 14-year-old old boy has had a recurrent cough associated with exercise for the past 6 months. The cough is episodic but has been worse since he joined the cross-country team. His medical history and results of a review of systems are unremarkable. Physical findings are normal. Which of the following is *most likely* to yield the correct diagnosis?

A) X-ray study of chest
B) Direct laryngoscopy
C) Nasal smear for eosionophils
D) Serum IgE concentration
E) Pulmonary function test

166) Which one of the following statements is true regarding the management of acute asthma exacerbations in children?

A) Inhaled anticholinergics should be routinely used in cases of severe asthma exacerbations
B) If a patient presents with fever they should be routinely started on antibiotics
C) A chest x-ray is helpful in all children experiencing an acute asthma exacerbation
D) Steroids improve pulmonary function compared with the use of bronchodilators alone with acute asthma
E) Studies show that nebulized albuterol is far superior to albuterol HFA with spacer use

Questions

167) Which of the following describes a patient with *mild persistent* asthma?

A) Symptoms more than 2 days a week but not daily and night symptoms no more than 2 times a month
B) Symptoms more than 2 days and nights a week
C) Symptoms more than 4 days and 4 nights a month
D) General symptoms greater than 2 times a month and night symptoms greater than 2 times a week
E) Symptoms more than 2 days a month and more than 2 nights a week

168) Each of the following is true regarding the management of children with persistent asthma *EXCEPT*:

A) Chronic use of inhaled steroids has a minimal, if any, impact on adult height
B) The risk of thrush from chronic inhaled steroid use can be minimized with the use of spacers and mouth rinsing after use
C) Chest x-rays in preschool children can be useful during acute exacerbations
D) Pulmonary function testing is the most objective measurement of status for preschool children
E) Children who have symptoms 4 days every week have moderate persistent asthma

169) Each of the following statements is true regarding pneumonia in children *EXCEPT*:

A) Its incidence is higher in children from lower socioeconomic levels
B) Boys have a higher incidence than girls
C) Fever and cough are the hallmark symptoms
D) Chest x-ray confirmation is needed before treatment can be instituted
E) Tachypnea is often a presenting sign.

Cardiology

170) Each of the following is a non-cardiac cause of chest pain *EXCEPT*:

A) Costochondritis
B) Anxiety
C) Exercise-induced asthma
D) Foreign body aspiration
E) Pleural effusion

171) Match the innocent murmur on the left with the description on the right.

1) Still's murmur
2) Pulmonary flow murmur
3) Cervical venous hum

(A) Systolic ejection-type murmur heard best over the upper left sternal border
(B) Low in pitch and often musical in quality
(C) Often present only when sitting or standing

172) An infant diagnosed with tetralogy of Fallot experiences a "hypercyanotic spell". Which one of the following would be *most appropriately* included in the management of this infant?

A) Subcutaneous morphine
B) Intramuscular phenobarbital
C) Oral Xanax® (alprazolam)
D) A trip to the Vulcan city of Xanadu
E) Intravenous calcium

Questions

173) A 7-year-old born with tricuspid atresia is sent to you because she is complaining of severe headaches coupled with vomiting for the past 3 days. She is afebrile and somewhat lethargic. Her physical examination her hematocrit is 53 and her WBC and the remainder of her labs are all normal. Which of the following is the MOST appropriate next diagnostic step?

A) Examination of CSF
B) Restriction of intake to clear fluids reexamination in 24 hours
C) X-ray study of the skull
D) Brain scan using technetium
E) Head CT

174) The parents of an asymptomatic 7-year-old boy with small VSD ask for your opinion regarding his participation in sports-related activities. Which of the following would be the MOST appropriate advice?

A) Contact sports should be avoided
B) Sustained isometric exercise should be avoided
C) Competitive track running is associated with an increased incidence of syncope
D) He can participate in all sports without additional cardiac risks
E) Activity should be restricted in high school, but limitations are unnecessary at this time

175) Which of the following drugs is MOST likely to be effective in *decreasing cardiac afterload* by decreasing systemic resistance?

A) Digoxin
B) Furosemide
C) Spironolactone
D) Chlorothiazide
E) Captopril

176) Syncope in a teenager brought on by which of the following is most ominous?

   A) Prolonged standing
   B) Exercise
   C) Headache
   D) Seizure
   E) Urination

177) The cardiac cath oxygen saturation and pressure gradient demonstrated below is most consistent with:

   A) Normal Heart
   B) Tetralogy of Fallot
   C) Total Anomalous venous return
   D) Pulmonary stenosis
   E) Aortic stenosis

	(SVC) 70%	(PV) 95%	
(RA)	2	5	(LA)
	70%	95%	
(RV)	22/2	110/10	(LV)
	70%	95%	
PA	30/15	110/70	A
	70%	95%	

Questions

178) You are evaluating a 16 year old high school varsity athlete whose 45 year old father is being treated for "high triglycerides or something like that" says the 16 year old.

Your athlete has recently been experiencing chest pain which radiates to the left shoulder and feels like pressure. On physical exam there is no abdominal pain and no chest pain with palpation. His blood pressure is 110/72 with no heart murmur noted.

The most appropriate step in managing this patient would be:

A) Trial of antacids no restrictions on playing ball
B) Abdominal CT with IV contrast to assess for cholecystitis
C) Trial of ibuprofen and no restrictions
D) EKG if not ST changes clear for full activity
E) Cardiology referral and restriction of sports and other strenuous exercise

179) Each of the following is seen in both simple atrioseptal defect and total anomalous venous return *EXCEPT:*

A) Palpable sternal lift
B) Tachypnea
C) Fixed splitting of S2
D) Cyanosis
E) Pulmonary flow murmur

Heme onc

180) Each of the following is associated with tumor lysis syndrome *EXCEPT*:

   A) Hyperphosphatemia
   B) Hyperkalemia
   C) Hypernatremia
   D) Hyperuricemia
   E) Alkalinization treatment

181) Each of the following is characteristic of Hodgkin's lymphoma *EXCEPT*:

   A) Reed-Sternberg cells
   B) Rapidly growing non-tender abdominal mass
   C) Non tender cervical nodes
   D) Elevated white blood cell count
   E) Low lymphocyte count

182) By definition, neutropenia in a 6 year old child is an absolute neutrophil count of less than:

   A) 400
   B) 1500
   C) 2500
   D) 3500
   E) 4500

183) A father with G6PD deficiency has a daughter who presented to the ER with dark urine. The girl is pale and lethargic. The BEST explanation for this is:

   A) Munchausen Syndrome by Proxy (MSBP)
   B) A new mutation
   C) Father is a carrier
   D) Mother is a carrier
   E) Father has the disorder and mom is a carrier

184) A 3 year old presents with a history of recurrent stomatitis, lymph node enlargement, and one episode of clostridium perfringens pneumonia. You suspect a diagnosis of cyclic neutropenia. What interval between neutropenic phases would help you confirm the diagnosis?

A) 1 week
B) 3 weeks
C) 24 weeks
D) 36 weeks
E) 6 months – 1 year
F) A millennium plus or minus a century

185) Please match the association on the left with the diagnosis on the right.

1) Lysosomal granules
2) Chronic Staph infections
3) Delayed separation of the umbilical stump
4) Clostridium perfringens
5) Pancreatic insufficiency

(A) Chediak-Hitachi syndrome
(B) Chronic granulomatous disease
(C) Cyclic neutropenia
(D) Leukocyte adhesion deficiency
(E) Shwachman-Diamond syndrome

186) In the following set of questions, decide if each numbered choice applies to (A) only, (B) only, both (C), or neither (D):

1) Low iron binding capacity
2) Low serum ferritin
3) High serum ferritin
4) Low MCV, low RDW

(A) Anemia of chronic illness
(B) Iron deficiency anemia
(C) Both
(D) Neither

187) In the following set of questions, decide if each numbered choice applies to (A) only, (B) only, both (C), or neither (D):

1) X-linked recessive
2) Autosomal dominant
3) Mucosal bleeds

(A) Hemophilia A
(B) Hemophilia B (Christmas disease)
(C) Both
(D) Neither

188) In the following set of questions, decide if each numbered choice applies to (A) only, (B) only, both (C), or neither (D):

    1) Uncommon in African Americans
    2) History of trauma
    3) Pain worse at night, relieved by ibuprofen
    4) Eats a lot of donuts, works in the safety department at a nuclear reactor and is cerebrally challenged

    (A) Ewing's sarcoma
    (B) Osteogenic sarcoma
    (C) Both
    (D) Neither

189) In the following set of questions, decide if each numbered choice applies to (A) only, (B) only, both (C), or neither (D):

    1) Normocytic anemia
    2) Macrocytic anemia
    3) Affects the red cell line primarily
    4) Primarily occurs in the newborn period
    5) Spontaneous recovery
    6) Primarily seen in toddlers

    (A) Transient erythroblastopenia of childhood
    (B) Diamond Blackfan syndrome
    (C) Both
    (D) Neither

190) A 1-year-old boy has been less active for the past 3-4 days with decreased appetite. With the exception of a URI 3 weeks earlier, he has done well. He is afebrile and his vital signs are stable. Except for notable pallor, the rest of the physical exam is unremarkable.

His labs include a WBC of 7.3, ANC of 100, H/H of 18/6, and MCV of 80. His platelet count is 352 K with a retic count of 0.1%. The MOST likely diagnosis is:

A) G6PD deficiency
B) Iron deficiency anemia
C) Diamond-Blackfan anemia
D) Alpha thalassemia
E) Transient erythroblastopenia of childhood

191) A 2-year-old boy is brought to you for an evaluation because he has been walking with an unsteady gait and occasionally exhibits "seizure-like activities" such as random eye movements and "myoclonic" movements. An abdominal mass is noted on physical examination.

The MOST likely preliminary diagnosis is:

A) Cerebral palsy
B) Trauma secondary to child abuse
C) Wilms' tumor
D) Neuroblastoma
E) Myoclonic seizure disorder

192) A 16-year-old girl is due to have a dental extraction. Her history is significant for menorrhagia and prolonged oozing following a similar dental procedure a year ago. Before going ahead with this procedure, one would be best advised to:

A) Administer platelets and fresh frozen plasma prior to the procedure
B) Have the dentist increase his coverage limits on her malpractice policy
C) Administer Factor VIII and titrate to achieve appropriate hemostasis
D) Before proceeding, do a coagulation workup to rule out von Willebrand's disease
E) Before proceeding, do a coagulation workup to rule out Factor VIII deficiency

193) A 3-year-old boy has been seen for chronic seborrheic dermatitis of the scalp of worsening severity. In addition, there is concern over polydipsia, polyuria, and discharge from his ear.[4] Realizing that this is not simply seborrheic dermatitis, you diagnose:

A) Seborrheic dermatitis with secondary infection
B) Severe combined immunodeficiency
C) Wiskott-Aldrich syndrome
D) Stevens-Johnson syndrome
E) Langerhans' cell histiocytosis

---

4 Poly otorrhea, if you will.

194) Which of the following conditions would be of MOST concern regarding malignant transformation?

A) Ichthyosis vulgaris
B) Strawberry hemangioma
C) Incontinentia pigmenti
D) Xeroderma pigmentosum
E) Acanthosis nigricans

195) Which of the following neoplasms shows the strongest familial tendency?

A) Osteosarcoma
B) Congenital hepatoma
C) Retinoblastoma
D) Wilms' tumor
E) Acute lymphoblastic leukemia

196) An 8-year-old boy with sickle cell disease has had abdominal pain, nausea, and vomiting for 8 hours. He has had similar pain intermittently over the past 5 months. He is afebrile, slightly jaundiced, and that there is upper quadrant abdominal tenderness. Which of the following is the MOST appropriate next step in evaluating this patient?

A) Upper gastrointestinal endoscopy
B) X-ray of the abdomen
C) Barium swallow
D) Ultrasound of the gallbladder
E) Exploratory laparotomy

197) The *most common* indication for a transfusion in a patient with hereditary spherocytosis would be:

A) Extramedullary hematopoiesis
B) Aplastic crisis
C) Severe fatigue
D) Hypersplenism
E) Growth retardation

Questions

198) Which of the following statements is true regarding the inheritance pattern of hereditary spherocytosis?

   A) It is primarily X linked recesssive
   B) It is primarily X linked dominant
   C) It is primarily autosomal recessive
   D) It is primarily autosomal dominant
   E) It is rarely seen in people of Northern European descent

199) Which of the following is true regarding splenectomy in children with hereditary spherocytosis?

   A) Partial splenectomy is of no benefit
   B) Splenectomy should be done prior to age 5 to be of any benefit
   C) Splenectomy is indicated for patients with splenomegaly before allowing them to participate in contact sports
   D) The risk of infection is highest one year after splenectomy
   E) Whenever possible, it's preferred over prophylactic penicillin

200) Treatment with which of the following chemotherapeutic agents increases the risk for developing bladder cancer as a *secondary malignancy*?

   A) Anthracycline
   B) Etoposide
   C) Ifosfamide
   D) Cyclophosphamide
   E) Methotrexate

201) The best way to confirm folate deficiency prior to treatment is by checking:

   A) Serum folate levels
   B) Mean corpuscle volume
   C) Segmented neutrophils
   D) Erythrocyte folic acid concentration
   E) Reticulocyte count

202) You are evaluating a patient who has hyperpigmented patches and is below the 10th percentile for both weight and height. On physical exam you also note that the patient has thumbs which can best be described as non-functional and small.

The most likely explanation for the findings would be:

A) Bloom syndrome
B) Rubinstein Taybi syndrome
C) Thrombocytopenia absent radius
D) Fanconi anemia
E) Osteogenic sarcoma

203) You are evaluating a 16 year old girl for intermittent right lower quadrant pain of 6 weeks duration. Her last menstrual period was 3 weeks ago. She denies sexual activity and her urine pregnancy test is negative. You order a pelvic ultrasound which reveals multiple ovarian cysts measuring less than 2 cm.

The most appropriate next step in managing this patient would be:

A) Obtain a Serum BHCG
B) Renal ultrasound
C) Amylase and lipase
D) Abdominal CT with oral and IV contrast
E) Serum tumor markers to rule out ovarian cancer

204) You are evaluating a 4-year-old boy with a 1 week history of a runny nose, cough and low grade fever. His appetite is decreased but he is taking in clear liquids with good urine output. His grandmother notes that he "never eats" and "doesn't weigh enough ". His immunizations are up to date. On examination you note clear nasal discharge and some irritated skin below and outside his nares. You also note a cluster of lymph nodes in the neck, which are pea sized and fully mobile with minimal tenderness. Growth and development have been unremarkable. Which of the following would be the most appropriate management:

A) Start antibiotics and a follow-up exam on lymph nodes in 2 weeks
B) Reassurance only
C) Biopsy lymph nodes
D) Thyroid function studies
E) PPD and chest X-ray

Renal

205) The mother of a 15-year-old has hypertension and has just been diagnosed with autosomal-dominant polycystic kidney disease. The child is asymptomatic. Physical findings and urine analysis are normal. Which of the following is the MOST appropriate next step in the evaluation of this child?

   A) MRI
   B) Renal US
   C) Repeat urinalysis and serum calcium levels
   D) Magnetic angiography (MRA)
   E) Urine creatinine clearance study

206) A 13-year-old boy is being followed for microscopic hematuria noted on several occasions over the past year. His history is negative and the family history reveals no evidence of renal disease or hematuria. His urinalysis shows 30 RBC/hpf and is negative for protein. Erythrocyte casts are noted. Serum creatinine and C3 are both normal. The urine calcium creatinine ratio as well as abdominal U/S are normal. Which of the following is the MOST appropriate next step?

   A) Voiding cystourethrogram
   B) Repeat the urine analysis in followup
   C) Renal biopsy
   D) IVP
   E) Abdominal CT

207) You note the following results on a urinalysis.

   Specific gravity of 1.023, pH of 5.5, Protein 2$^+$, negative for blood, WBC 0-4, RBC 0-3, epithelial cells 3-5, and bacteria – few. The history and physical exam are unremarkable. The MOST appropriate next step would be:

   A) Obtain a renal ultrasound
   B) Obtain a first AM urine protein/creatinine ratio
   C) Obtain serum BUN, creatinine, liver function tests, and serum albumin
   D) Urine culture and presumptive treatment with trimethoprim-sulfamethoxazole
   E) Obtain a 24-hour urine protein

208) Low serum C_3 levels are seen with each of the following *EXCEPT*:

A) Focal segmental glomerulonephritis
B) Membranoproliferative glomerulonephritis
C) Acute post strep glomerulonephritis
D) Lupus nephritis
E) Shunt nephritis

209) You are evaluating an otherwise healthy 6-year-old child for nocturnal enuresis. All of the following can be associated with nocturnal enuresis *EXCEPT*:

A) Diabetes insipidus
B) Sickle cell disease
C) Seizure disorder
D) SIADH
E) Lumbosacral anomaly

210) Each of the following is a true statement regarding hemolytic uremic syndrome *EXCEPT*:

A) It occurs primarily during the summer months
B) It affects primarily pre-schoolers
C) Has a predilection for families of lower socioeconomic status
D) Has a predilection for families of higher socioeconomic status
E) Occurs more commonly in the Northern US and Canada

211) Which of the following types of renal stones form only in the setting of infection?

A) Calcium oxalate
B) Struvite
C) Uric acid
D) Cystine
E) Rolling

212) A child with inflammatory bowel disease develops a renal stone. Which of the following stone would be most likely?

A) Oxalate
B) Struvite
C) Uric Acid
D) Cystine
E) Mick Jagger

213) Which of the following constitute first line therapy for patients with hematuria and renal stones due to hypercalciuria?

A) Thiazide diuretics
B) Increase water intake
C) Low sodium diet
D) Alkalinization of urine
E) B and C

214) In addition to hematuria which of the following additional findings would raise the concern for a progressive renal disease?

A) Red cast cells
B) White blood cells
C) Proteinuria
D) Abdominal pain
E) Fever

215) You are evaluating a 4 year old with mild proteinuria, and a fever of 101.2 over the past 3 days. Her CBC is within normal limits.

   The most appropriate management at this time would be:

   A) Renal ultrasound
   B) Renal biopsy
   C) 24 hour urine creatinine collection
   D) One time measure of urine creatinine
   E) Repeat urine analysis in 3 weeks

216) Each of the following is an adverse effect of ACE inhibitors in children *EXCEPT*:

   A) Hypokalemia
   B) Neutropenia
   C) Angioedema
   D) Dry cough
   E) Anemia

217) Each of the following are associated with a false proteinuria on urine dipstick *EXCEPT*:

   A) Chlorhexidine wipe contamination
   B) Gross hematuria
   C) Alkaline pH
   D) Urine specific gravity lower than 1.015
   E) Phenazopyridine

Genitourinary

218) A 4-year-old girl is having difficulty with toilet training. The parents report that their daughter has constant dribbling of urine during the day and night. On examination, urine appears to be draining from the vagina. Results of urine analysis and culture are normal. Which of the following is the MOST likely diagnosis?

   A) Diabetes insipidus
   B) Neurogenic bladder
   C) Giggling incontinence
   D) UTI
   E) Ectopic uretal orifice

219) A 17-year-old boy had a unilateral orchidopexy for a cryptorchid testis when he was 10 years old. He now seeks further information. You would tell him most appropriately that:

   A) Retractile testicles without intervention can result in cryptorchidism
   B) Surgical correction clearly decreases the overall risk of malignancy
   C) Self-examination of the testes on a regular basis is particularly important post-op
   D) Boys with a retractile testis are at increased risk for infertility or malignancy
   E) There is no cause for concern because operative correction was successful

220) You are evaluating a 2 month old boy for his routine physical exam. The baby's development has been progressing nicely; he is in the 50th percentile for height, weight and head circumference. The father who is in the 95th percentile for bad taste in T shirts and jeans is very concerned about the size of his son's penis. You measure the boy's penis and note it to be 4.1 centimeters and both testes are descended.

   The most appropriate next step in managing this patient would be:

   A) Ask the father why the obsession with his son's penis size
   B) Obtain a CT scan of the head
   C) Obtain a genetic karyotype
   D) Measure serum 17-hydroxy progesterone
   E) Delicately reassure the father

221) During a routine physical examination of an 18 month old you are unable to palpate the left testicle despite the documentation of bilateral descended testicle during previous visits.

The most appropriate next step in evaluating this patient would be:

A) Testicular ultrasound
B) Trial of HCG shots
C) Urological consult
D) Reposition and re-examine the patient
E) Transilluminate the scrotum

222) A 16-year-old girl presents to the Emergency Department at 1:00 AM reporting that she has had intermittent mild abdominal pain and nausea for 10 days. Her physical exam is unremarkable. UA reveals Sp. gravity of 1.010, a trace of glucose, no protein, and 2-3 WBC/HPF. The MOST appropriate next step would be to order:

A) An abdominal CT
B) Barium enema
C) IVP
D) Urine human chorionic gonadotropin
E) Glucose tolerance test

223) Which of the following is true regarding acute testicular pain?

A) The blue dot sign is commonly seen in testicular torsion
B) Torsion of the testicular appendage requires immediate surgical excision
C) Nausea and vomiting are the hallmarks of epididymitis
D) True bacterial epididymitis is rare in children
E) Inguinal hernia never results in acute scrotal pain

224) You are evaluating a 17-year-old boy who is concerned about a lump on his testicle. He notes that the pain varies from sharp to dull discomfort and denies any trauma. The lump is more noticeable when he stands and is less noticeable when he lies down. Which of the following is the most likely diagnosis?

A) Seminoma
B) Inguinal hernia
C) Hydrocele
D) Varicocele
E) Normal finding

Neurology

225) While you are on rounds, a child is presented with acute lateralized weakness and, since you haven't slept since the first season of American Idol®, your "differential" is limited to "acute stroke". The attending physician is appalled and asks you to do 5 pushups over a bedpan suspended by a fish line held by the medical students. With each pushup, you are to shout each diagnosis in the differential. You will have redeemed yourself if you call out each of the following **EXCEPT**:

   A) Todd postictal paralysis
   B) Hemiparetic seizures
   C) Subdural hemorrhage
   D) Hypocalcemia
   E) Hypoglycemia

226) A 10 month old presents with rapid onset hypotonia, lethargy and constipation. Mom states that no new foods have been introduced into the infant's diet. On physical exam, you also note mydriasis and diminished reflexes. This condition would *BEST* be diagnosed with:

   A) Head CT
   B) Head MRI
   C) Karyotype
   D) Tensilon test
   E) EMG

227) Primary treatment for the above diagnosis would be:

   A) Gentamicin
   B) Tensilon
   C) Ampicillin and ceftriaxone
   D) Immunization update
   E) Supportive

228) A 6 year old girl with mild intellectual disability and a history of infantile spasms presents with new seizures. On physical exam, you note microcephaly and several hypopigmented patches distributed over her body along with a fleshy bump near her nose. This disorder would *BEST* be diagnosed with which study?

A) Head CT
B) Head MRI
C) Karyotype
D) EEG
E) EMG

229) In the following set of questions, decide if each numbered choice applies to (A) only, (B) only, both (C), or neither (D):

1) Can involve the eyes
2) Progressive onset
3) Treatment is curative
4) Prevented with immunization

(A) Infantile botulism
(B) Myasthenia gravis
(C) Both
(D) Neither

230) Match the diagnosis on the left with the clinical history on the right.

1) Structural headaches
2) Migraine
3) Tension headache

(A) Pain in the neck or shoulders
(B) Aggravated by sneezing, coughing, or straining
(C) Cyclic vomiting and recurrent abdominal pain

231) A 10-year-old boy was diagnosed with migraine headaches one year ago. His headaches have been treated with ibuprofen. Over the past few weeks he has been complaining of early morning headaches, often severe enough to wake him up. There has been a lot of academic pressure at school according to the parents. He has also vomited before breakfast in the morning.

On physical examination, you note that his fundi are normal and that he has mild lower extremity hyperreflexia. The gait is normal and tone and strength are equal and symmetric. Which of the following is the MOST appropriate next step?

A) Order MRI of the head
B) Order an EEG
C) Refer to a psychologist for anxiety management
D) Suggest eating breakfast first thing in the morning
E) Consider beta blockers to control performance anxiety rather than ibuprofen

232) In an average full term newborn, whose parent have average sized heads, a head circumference of 40 cm would be considered:

A) Macrocephaly
B) Microcephaly
C) Craniosynostosis
D) Normocephalic
E) Beckwith-Wiedemann syndrome

233) You are presented with an infant who is exhibiting a multifocal clonic seizure. Attempts to control it with phenobarbital have failed. You review the EEG tracing and stroke your beardless chin.[5] You appear to be concentrating deeply even though, to your untrained eye, the EEG looks no different than the geological society tracing of a typical earthquake. However, Lenny, your neurology consultant informs you that it is a "paroxysmal pattern of generalized bursts of bilaterally synchronous high-voltage activity intermixed with spikes or short waves". The MOST likely explanation for these clinical findings and the EEG tracing would be:

A) Herpetic encephalitis
B) Confirmation of your suspicion that Lenny is a fraud, since this actually was a geological tracing of an earthquake you showed him
C) Pyridoxine dependency
D) Hypoxic-ischemic encephalopathy
E) Intracranial hemorrhage

234) A 3-month-old unimmunized infant newly adopted from overseas is noted to develop constipation and weakness over 5 days. He is alert but has drooping eyelids, sluggishly reactive pupils, and decreased reflexes. Findings on physical exam are otherwise normal. Which of the following is the *most likely* diagnosis?

A) Myasthenia gravis
B) Muscular dystrophy
C) Spinal muscular atrophy (Werdnig-Hoffmann disease)
D) Poliomyelitis
E) Infantile botulism

---

5 We are referring to female physicians here of course.

235) You are evaluating a 10 year old girl who has been experiencing headaches for the past few weeks. The headaches are primarily occipital accompanied by a spinning sensation, ringing sound, double vision and difficulty maintaining balance.

The headaches occur several times per week and in between headaches she is asymptomatic. The neurological exam is unremarkable.

Which of the following is the most likely diagnosis?

A) Conversion disorder.
B) Posterior fossa tumor
C) Viral labyrinthitis
D) Basilar type migraine
E) Familial hemiplegic migraine

236) Each of the following is a recommendation to reduce the frequency and severity of migraine headaches *EXCEPT*:

A) Regular sleep
B) Exercise
C) Elimination diets
D) Biofeedback
E) Stress management

237) You are caring for a 5 year old child who has been experiencing daily headaches over his left eye. He is not experiencing any nausea or vomiting, ataxia, visual or hearing deficits. He has been taking acetaminophen and ibuprofen several times a day with no relief. Other than a minor head trauma 6 weeks ago with no loss of consciousness, there is no history of trauma.

The most likely cause of the chronic headaches would be:

A) Subdural hematoma
B) Epidural hematoma
C) Medication overuse headaches
D) Basilar type migraine
E) Familial hemiplegic migraine

238) You are caring for an 8 year old boy who was noted by the teachers to be periodically staring out the window without responding to her snapping her finger. Occasional facial twitching occurs during these episodes. Which of the following would be the most appropriate treatment for this child?

A) Methylphenidate
B) Atomoxetine
C) Desipramine
D) Lamotrigine
E) Carbamazepine

239) Each of the following would constitute appropriate treatment of infantile spasms *EXCEPT*:

A) Ketogenic diet
B) Carbamazepine
C) Adrenocorticotropic hormone
D) Valproic acid
E) Topiramate

240) Each of the following medications would be appropriate for treating generalized, non-focal, non-absence seizure in children *EXCEPT*:

A) Phenytoin
B) Valproic acid
C) Lamotrigine
D) Topiramate
E) Levetiracetam

241) Which of the following would be most appropriate for treating complex partial seizures in children?

   A) Ethosuximide
   B) Valproic Acid
   C) Carbamazepine
   D) Phenobarbital
   E) Phenytoin

242) Which of the following would be appropriate for treating primary absence seizures in children?

   A) Ethosuximide
   B) Valproic Acid
   C) Carbamazepine
   D) Phenobarbital
   E) Phenytoin

Musculoskeletal

243) A frantic mother and her neighbor bring a 2 1/2 year old to your office in an ambulance. She has had hip pain for the past 2-3 days but does not appear to be ill. You comfort the child by giving her a stuffed Spongebob Squarepants doll.

While examining her you are able to move her hip through some flexion and abduction. She has a fever of 38.1°C, and the mother notes that she recently had a cold. Lab results include a WBC of 11.2 with an ESR of 22. The ultrasound report indicates fluid in the affected hip. You suggest:

A) Urgent orthopedic consultation for drainage and culture of fluid
B) Bone scan
C) Rest, reassurance, ibuprofen and outpatient follow-up
D) Oral antibiotics and close follow up
E) Admit to the hospital for IV antibiotics

244) A 3 year old boy brought to your office. His father, who at first glance appears to actually have no neck, requests braces because his kid is "walking like a pigeon" and will interfere with his football career. He notes that he had the same problem and had bars every night and this "set him straight". You suggest:

A) The father seek counseling and Prolixin Decanoate intramuscular IM for one month under psychiatric supervision
B) Ballet classes for father and son, and laughingly suggest no "bars" are needed, including the ones the father apparently visits on a nightly basis.
C) Denis-Browne bars every night to correct this problem that should have resolved by 18 months
D) Reassurance that the problem with resolve with time without the aid of bars and devices
E) A referral to physical therapy

245) A newborn male is noted to have disproportionately short limbs as well as a small chest. He has multiple healed fractures as well as new fractures of the long bones and ribs. Which of the following disorders would account for these findings?

A) Achondrogenesis
B) Trifecta imperfecta
C) Thanatophoric dysplasia
D) Juvenile osteochondroses
E) Osteogenesis imperfecta

246) A 2-year-old presents to the ED because of refusal to use his left arm. The child is afebrile with no evidence of trauma on physical examination. The left elbow is noted to be flexed, with the forearm in a pronated position. There is no swelling or discoloration, although the child is reluctant to allow you to examine the arm. The MOST appropriate next step is to:

A) Order and x-ray of the elbow
B) Order a bone scan
C) Check a CBC, blood culture, and start antibiotics
D) Apply a splint and refer to ortho
E) Supinate the forearm while the elbow is flexed

247) A 13-year-old boy is sent to you by his coach because of pain and swelling below his left knee. He is active in sports, particularly running, baseball, and skiing. Physical examination reveals joint tenderness over the anterior tubercle of the left knee. Which of the following is the most likely diagnosis?

A) Patellar dislocation
B) Osteochondritis dissecans
C) Tear of the collateral ligament
D) Osgood-Schlatter disease
E) Tear of medial meniscus

248) A 12-year-old girl has a 7-week history of pain in the right heel. For the past 4 weeks she has also had pain in the left heel, the left calf, and the Achilles tendon. The pain worsens with walking.

The patient has been excused from all physical activity at school, including opening and closing her locker. She now refuses to walk, claiming that her leg is "paralyzed." She is afebrile and presents with no other symptoms.

On physical examination, the patient appears to be well but is somewhat uncomfortable and frequently shifts her position while seated but cannot move the left leg. Muscle tone and reflexes of the left leg are normal; the leg can be moved passively without pain or discomfort. Physical exam is otherwise unremarkable. Of the following, the most appropriate next step in the evaluation of this patient's condition would be to:

A) Begin administration of nonsteroidal inflammatory drugs
B) Measure antinuclear antibody titers
C) Order x-ray studies of both lower extremities
D) Elicit additional history
E) Obtain an electromyogram

249) Osteomyelitis can spread locally to cause septic arthritis. After which age does is this risk reduced?

A) 6 months
B) 12 months
C) 36 months
D) 48 months
E) closure of the growth plate

250) Which of the following differentiates clubfoot from metatarsus adductus?

A) Putting your foot in your mouth (figuratively of course)
B) Inability to dorsiflex the ankle with metatarsus adductus
C) Inability to dorsiflex the ankle with club foot
D) Positive Babinski with club foot
E) Negative Babinski with club foot

251) The definition of scoliosis is:

   A) A spinal curvature greater than 10 degrees on a posterior-anterior x-ray
   B) A spinal curvature greater than 10 degrees on an anterior-posterior x-ray
   C) A spinal curvature greater than 25 degrees on a posterior-anterior x-ray
   D) A spinal curvature greater than 25 degrees on an anterior-posterior x-rays
   E) Based on clinical findings and pulmonary function

252) Duchenne muscular dystrophy is due to the absence of dystrophin which results in:

   A) Muscle membrane instability
   B) Nerve transmission disfunction
   C) Neuromuscular junction blockade
   D) Increased acetylcholine presynaptic uptake
   E) Replacement of dystrophin with collagen

253) You are caring for a family where there is a child with Duchenne muscular dystrophy. There is no prior family history and the molecular genetic testing in the child is negative. The risk for recurrence is closest to:

   A) 0%
   B) 10%
   C) 25%
   D) 90%
   E) 100%

254) Congenital talipes equinovarus (club foot) is typically diagnosed by:

   A) Cribside clinical diagnosis
   B) CT scan
   C) MRI
   D) Ultrasound
   E) Bone Scan

255) If conservative measures to treat congenital talipes equinovarus (club foot) are unsuccessful, when should surgical interventions be implemented?

   A) When the child begins to walk
   B) When the child enters school
   C) During pubertal development
   D) During the first year of life
   E) When the growth plates fuse

256) When ruling out a muscular based disorder in a patient who is hypotonic which of the following would be the most appropriate initial screening test to order?

   A) Serum anti-nuclear antibody level (ANA)
   B) Double stranded DNA measurement
   C) Serum creatinine kinase measurement
   D) EMG of the lower extremity
   E) Muscle Biopsy

Dermatology

257) The cutaneous manifestation seen in rheumatic fever is:

   A) Erythema multiforme
   B) Erythema marginatum
   C) Erythema nodosum
   D) Erythema migrans
   E) Erythema infectiosum

258) In the following set of questions, for each numbered word or phrase, choose the lettered heading that is MOST CLOSELY ASSOCIATED with it. Lettered headings may be selected once, more than once, or not at all.

   1) May involve the mucous membranes
   2) Parvovirus B19
   3) Rash seen in 70% of cases of Lyme disease
   4) Associated with inflammatory bowel disease
   5) Eyes glazed over trying to determine which erythema is correct on the Exam-ema
   6) Erythematous macules on the back

   (A) Erythema marginatum
   (B) Erythema nodosum
   (C) Erythema infectiosum
   (D) Erythema multiforme
   (E) Erythema migrans
   (F) Erythema confusiosum

259) Which of the following dermatological manifestations is seen with tuberculosis?

   A) Erythema confusiosum
   B) Erythema multiforme
   C) Erythema nodosum
   D) Erythema migrans
   E) Erythema infectiosum

Questions

260) Which of the following lesions is most consistently found on children with tuberous sclerosis?

A) Cafe au lait spot
B) Periungual fibromas
C) Sclerosing tubers
D) Port wine stains
E) Ash leaf macules

261) A 6-week-old formula-fed infant presents with a progressively worsening rash. The rash is observed in the axilla, neck, and the diaper area and appears to be yellowish, greasy, and scaly, but non-pruritic. The mother is very concerned; all attempts to treat with "previously prescribed creams" and lotions have not helped. The MOST appropriate next step in managing this infant and the mother's concerns would be:

A) Reassurance
B) Zinc supplement
C) Switching the infant to an elemental formula
D) Oral prednisone
E) Referral to Dermatology for skin biopsy

262) A 3-month-old former 32-week premie presents with crusty plaques around the mouth and on the face. The plaques have distinct margins. In addition, the infant is irritable and has patches of missing hair and moderate diarrhea. The BEST step in managing this patient would be:

A) Reassurance
B) Zinc supplements
C) Hydrocortisone cream and nystatin ointment
D) Moisturizing lotions and soap
E) Skin biopsy

263) Match the lettered diagnosis on the right with the description on the left.

1) Inflammation and black dots
2) Complete areas of smooth hair loss
3) Incomplete patches of hair loss
4) Eyebrows are typically involved
5) Pediatrician preparing for the boards

(A) Alopecia totalis
(B) Alopecia areata
(C) Tinea capitis
(D) Alopecia neurotica
(E) Trichotillomania

264) A 4-year-old girl is being seen for "infected mosquito bites" on the lower part of her leg. She is also noted to have "puffy" eyelids. The rest of her physical exam is normal. Which of the following would be the most appropriate next step?

A) Culture of the material scraped from the skin lesions
B) CBC and ESR
C) Urinalysis
D) Prescription of Pen VK and reexamination in one week
E) Hospitalization

265) A 15-year-old girl has a one-week history of pruritic rash on her back and chest. The rash started with one "spot" approximately 2 cm in size on her chest. She is taking no medication and has no other significant medical history. Physical examination reveals an afebrile patient with a diffuse, hyperpigmented, papular rash on her back and chest. Which of the following is the most likely diagnosis?

A) Pityriasis rosea
B) Psoriasis
C) Keratosis pilaris
D) Lyme disease
E) Parvovirus infection

266) Each of the following conditions is associated with the production of an exotoxin *EXCEPT*:

   A) Scarlet fever
   B) Hemolytic uremic syndrome
   C) Toxic shock syndrome
   D) Toxic epidermal necrolysis
   E) Staphylococcal scalded skin syndrome

267) A 13-month-old has an excoriated rash about the neck, wrists, ankles, and genitalia. His mother has a similar pruritic rash. Which of the following is the most definitive therapy for this condition?

   A) Topical application of corticosteroids
   B) Systemic administration of antihistamines
   C) Topical application of 5% permethrin cream
   D) Systemic administration of corticosteroids
   E) Typical application of wet dressings with Burow's solution

Rheumatology

268) All of the following are considered major Jones criteria *EXCEPT*:

   A) Arthralgia and erythema chronicum migrans
   B) Carditis
   C) Arthritis and erythema marginatum
   D) Chorea
   E) Subcutaneous nodules

269) All of the following are true with regards to Kawasaki disease *EXCEPT*:

   A) It is more common among Asian populations
   B) It is more common among girls
   C) It is more prevalent in the winter and spring
   D) Most cases occur in children between 8 and 10 years of age
   E) IV gamma globulin given in the acute phase reduces the risk for coronary artery disease

270) All of the following are associated with Henoch Schönlein purpura *EXCEPT*:

   A) IgA nephropathy
   B) Proteinuria
   C) Hematuria
   D) Thrombocytopenia
   E) Anaphylactoid purpura

Questions

271) An 8 year old boy reports to your office complaining of 2 weeks of lack of energy and just not feeling like playing with the other kids. He has had a persistent low-grade fever.

On physical exam, you see that his throat is non-injected, his TMs are clear, and there is no nasal discharge. His lungs are clear and you note a systolic ejection click heard best at the apex. Abdominal exam reveals a non-tender abdomen, soft with no guarding or rebound, no hepatomegaly but 2 – 3 cm. splenomegaly. He has no significant joint aches; however, you do note some tenderness over the pads of his fingers. The best study to confirm this diagnosis would be:

- A) Abdominal CT and serological studies
- B) Bone scan
- C) Blood culture
- D) Cardiac echo and chest X ray
- E) IV Ig based on your presumptive diagnosis, with close follow-up of signs of coronary arterial dilation

272) Each of the following would be suggestive of a new case of rheumatic fever *EXCEPT*:

- A) Nonspecific pink macules that cover the trunk, prolonged PR interval, arthralgia, and a positive throat culture for group A beta hemolytic strep
- B) A marked deterioration in their handwriting, emotional lability
- C) Firm, non-tender, pea-sized nodules on knees and elbows and over the spine
- D) Pericardial effusion, with first-degree heart block
- E) High, spiking fever for 6 days, bilateral conjunctivitis, skin peeling noted on the fingers

273) Each of the following is a clinical manifestation of Kawasaki disease *EXCEPT*:

- A) Thrombocytosis
- B) Bacterial meningitis
- C) Sterile pyuria
- D) Hydrops of the gallbladder
- E) Conjunctivitis

274) Which one of the following is associated with systemic lupus erythematosus?

A) Conjunctivitis
B) Erythema chronicum migrans
C) Erythema multiforme
D) Palmar erythema
E) Erythema marginatum

275) In patients with systemic lupus erythematosus, which organ system is likely to cause the most serious morbidity and mortality?

A) Hematological
B) Central nervous system
C) Renal
D) Cardiac
E) It is too variable to determine

276) Which one of the following maternal serum antibodies is most associated with congenital heart block in a newborn?

A) ANA
B) Anti –Sm. (Smith)
C) Anti-ds DNA
D) Anti-Ro
E) Anti-La

277) Which of the following is true regarding the epidemiology of systemic lupus erythematosus?

A) African –Americans are the most susceptible racial group to develop lupus
B) Only 5% of all patients who have lupus are diagnosed in childhood
C) After puberty, the female to male ratio drops down to 2:1
D) Prior to puberty, the female to male ratio is 3:1
E) Most pediatric patients are diagnosed prior to puberty

278) Which of the following is the most common presenting sign of early localized Lyme disease?

A) Single erythema migrans rash at the site of the tick bite
B) Multiple disseminated erythema migrans rash
C) Myalgia
D) Headache
E) Fatigue

279) Each of the following are commonly seen in Kawasaki disease (KD) *EXCEPT*:

A) Discreet oral ulcers and tonsillar exudate
B) Bilateral non-exudative conjunctivitis
C) Diffusely erythematous oropharynx
D) Red Fissured lips
E) Strawberry tongue

Ophthalmology

280) You are evaluating a 3 year old boy who has just started preschool. The teacher has noted that he often lifts his chin to see material on the board. On examination you note that the left eyelid is a bit lower than the right. His pupils are equal and reactive with extraocular eye movements intact and unremarkable.

The most likely explanation for this would be:

A) Behavioral
B) Vernal conjunctivitis
C) Congenital amblyopia
D) Congenital ptosis
E) Horner syndrome

281) You are evaluating a 3 year old boy who has just started preschool. The teacher has noted that he often lifts his chin to see material on the board. On examination you note that the right eyelid is a bit lower than the left. His right pupil is slower to react to light than the left. You note that the left side of his hair is matted while the right seems to be soft and light. The parents laugh and note that is how he got the nickname "left sweat head".

The most likely diagnosis is:

A) Kings lead hat syndrome
B) Congenital ptosis
C) Myasthenia gravis
D) Amblyopia
E) Horner syndrome

282) Which of the following is associated with congenital cataracts?

A) Lactase deficiency
B) Maternal hypoparathyroidism
C) Maternal hypothyroidism
D) Maternal hyperthyroidism
E) Maternal hyperparathyroidism

283) A 4 year old girl presents to your office unable to fully open her right eye. You note that the eye has tearing and the upper eyelid is pink with mild swelling. She was on a camp trip to the beach when she complained of her right eye hurting. She was okay this morning when she woke up and no discharge was noted. She is afebrile and her immunizations are up to date. When you apply topical tetracaine she was able to open her eye and was less apprehensive. No FB was seen on closer exam, and under fluorescein staining there was a 5mm area of increased uptake on the edge of the cornea. Which of the following would be the most appropriate next step?

   A) Application of pressure patch overnight
   B) Gentamicin ophthalmic eye drops without pressure patch
   C) Erythromycin ophthalmic ointment with pressure patch
   D) Erythromycin ophthalmic ointment without pressure patch
   E) Immediate ophthalmology consultation

284) You are evaluating a 3 week old infant with excessive tearing since birth and few days of mucoid discharge noted on the left eye. The tears appear to trickle down the eyelid to the left cheek. The conjunctiva is mildly injected. Neonatal history is unremarkable and erythromycin ointment was applied at the time of delivery. There is no history of cough, difficulty feeding or fever at this time. . Which of the following would the most appropriate management?

   A) Immediate ophthalmological consultation for evaluation and management of gonococcal conjunctivitis
   B) Immediate hospital admission for treatment of Chlamydia conjunctivitis
   C) Instructing the mother on massage technique to unblock tear duct
   D) Application of erythromycin ophthalmic ointment 4 times a day
   E) Oral erythromycin 4 times a day

ENT

285) A healthy 8 month old presents to your office with stridor that worsens with inspiration and improves with expiration. You explain to the parents that:

A) Surgical correction will be needed
B) Direct laryngoscopy will be needed
C) A barium swallow is indicated to rule out extrinsic compression
D) No intervention is necessary at this time because this condition will improve with time
E) They should consider a career in "creative" yodeling for the child

286) The diagnosis of otitis media is BEST made through:

A) Mothers' insistence on antibiotics because they are leaving on a trip
B) Tympanometry
C) Pneumatic otoscopy
D) A dull tympanic membrane
E) Audiometry

287) All of the following are true statements regarding airway obstruction "above the glottis" <u>EXCEPT</u>:

A) "Hot potato" voice can be a sign
B) Obstruction improves with expiration
C) It can present as a surgical emergency
D) It typically presents with expiratory stridor
E) High fever and drooling can be a feature

Questions

288) A 3-year-old boy has a fever of 39.8C and severe respiratory distress. Three days prior to this present illness, he developed rhinorrhea, a brassy cough, and a low-grade fever.

On physical examination, he has stridor and retractions along with decreased air entry. Oxygen saturation is 90%. Lateral x-ray of the neck shows a normal epiglottis. AP views show a "shaggy" border of the tracheal air shadow. The MOST likely diagnosis is:

A) Bacterial tracheitis
B) Acute spasmodic croup
C) Viral croup
D) Foreign body aspiration
E) Croupier disease

289) The best treatment for the above condition would include:

A) Dexamethasone
B) Racemic epinephrine
C) Cool mist
D) IV fluids
E) IV antibiotics

290) Each of the following is true regarding laryngotracheitis *EXCEPT*:

A) It is also known as "viral croup"
B) Most cases occur in the early spring or late fall
C) Typical age of patient is 12 months
D) It has an abrupt onset with no preceding upper respiratory infection
E) Stridor is biphasic

291) You have in your practice a healthy fully-immunized toddler with acute otitis media with effusion. The father is a microbiologist and he wants to know the likely etiology. You would be correct in telling him that it is likely to be any of the following *EXCEPT*:

A) Haemophilus influenza type B
B) Adenovirus
C) Streptococcus pneumoniae
D) Moraxella catarrhalis
E) Parainfluenza virus

292) Each of the following is true regarding laryngeal papillomas *EXCEPT*:

   A) Laser excision often needs to be repeated
   B) Radiation treatment reduces the risk for malignant degeneration
   C) It is acquired at birth from maternal vaginal condylomata
   D) Surgery is not curative
   E) They are not considered to be true neoplasm

293) You are seeing a child for persistent middle ear effusion following two episodes of otitis media treated with antibiotics. Which of the following is true regarding the middle ear effusion?

   A) Inflammatory mediators play a role
   B) Decreased blood flow to the mucous membranes is a factor
   C) It is most likely due to persistent infection
   D) Engorgement secondary to allergies is the likely cause
   E) It may eventually require myringotomy tube placement

294) A 7-year-old previously healthy girl presents with a postauricular mass of 9 months' duration. The mass is firm, non-tender. She is afebrile and there is and has been no erythema or any other neck masses. The MOST likely etiology is:

   A) Psychogenic adenopathy
   B) Atypical mycobacteria
   C) Cat scratch fever
   D) Neoplastic disease
   E) Paramyxovirus

295) You are the attending in the ER, where you are presented with a 6-year-old boy with a 4-hour history of inspiratory stridor and a temperature of 38.1C. The parents have refused immunizations out of concern for the "increased risk for autoimmune disease". The child is apprehensive and leaning forward to facilitate breathing and you note that the child is also drooling. The MOST appropriate initial step would be to:

A) Obtain a lateral view x-ray study of the neck
B) Administer cefuroxime, 50 mg/kg IV
C) Request the presence of an individual skilled in intubation
D) Obtain an ABG
E) Examine the pharynx

296) Each of the following is true statements regarding acute otitis media *EXCEPT*:

A) Daily antibiotic prophylaxis is a proven method to prevent recurrent otitis
B) The pneumococcal vaccine has resulted in a drop in the incidence of OM due to S. pneumoniae
C) Exposure to passive smoke increases risk for recurrent OM
D) Children attending child care at increased risk for recurrent OM
E) Tympanostomy tubes are the treatment of choice for recurrent otitis media

297) Which of the following would be an appropriate antibiotic to use for a dental infection in a 4 year old patient who is allergic to penicillin?

A) Trimethoprim-sulfamethoxazole
B) Ciprofloxacin
C) Amoxicillin/Clavulanic acid
D) Clindamycin
E) Metronidazole

298) Which of the following should alert the clinician to an intracranial complication of otitis media?

   A) Hearing loss
   B) Otorrhea
   C) Otalgia
   D) Vomiting and blurred vision
   E) Rhinorrhea

299) Immediate treatment of focal swelling, pain and erythema of the pinna following a traumatic event consists of:

   A) Ice packs
   B) Application of a tight compress
   C) Prompt initiation of antibiotics
   D) Head CT
   E) Evacuation of hematoma

300) Which of the following pathogens is the most likely cause of chronic sinusitis?

   A) S. pneumoniae
   B) H. Flu type b
   C) Staph aureus
   D) Moraxella catarrhalis
   E) Group B strep

301) The SNAP[6] protocol has been used successfully to allow an ear infection to go 48 hours before parents will fill a prescription for antibiotics. Which of the following situations would prevent you from implementing this strategy?

   A) Fever for 24 hours
   B) Symptoms of otitis media for 24 hours
   C) Another episode of otitis media in the past 3 months
   D) Children younger than 18 months
   E) No movement of tympanic membrane with insufflation

---

6 Safety –net antibiotic prescription is what SNAP stands for.

302) A child with recurrent otitis media presents to your office. She has had several episodes of pneumonia requiring hospitalization. Growth and development are normal. On physical exam there are no oral lesions, lungs are clear, and heart sounds are normal with no thrills, murmur, or gallops, and you notice her heart sounds are loudest on the right side.

Which of the following would be most helpful in establishing a diagnosis?

A) Cardiac echo
B) Measurement of serum immunoglobulin levels
C) Sweat test
D) Electron microscopic examination of nasal mucosa
E) HIV testing

303) **Which of the following statements is true regarding treatment of upper respiratory tract infection caused by rhinovirus?**

A) Menthol improves nasal airflow and patency
B) Nasal congestion and sore throat improve with saline washes
C) Oseltamivir is effective if used within 48 hours of onset of symptoms
D) Guaifenesin increases cough frequency and clearance
E) Inhalation of steam reduces rhinovirus replication and viral titers in nasal secretions

304) You are evaluating a 9-year-old girl who presents with a tick that is attached to the back of her neck. The tick is moderately engorged and you successfully remove it and place it in a small vial. The parents are concerned since they live in a wooded area and have a neighbor who never recovered from Lyme disease. The most appropriate next step would be to:

A) Advise them to have all the trees in the area leveled with Napalm®
B) Prescribe Augmentin 50mg/kg/d in 3 divided doses for 14 days
C) Prescribe Amoxicillin 50 mg/kg/ in 3 divided doses for 21 days
D) Obtain ELISA / Western blot testing in 3 weeks
E) Reassure the parents that the risk for Lyme disease is quite low

305) You are evaluating a 17 year old girl with a 1 week history of clear rhinorrhea, intermittent sneezing and irritated red skin around her nose. She is afebrile and otherwise asymptomatic. She is not sexually active, menstrual periods are regular and she is not taking oral contraceptive pills. On examination, you note swollen blue turbinates. Her growth and development are unremarkable. Nasal smear is negative. She has not been taking any medications. The most likely diagnosis would be:

A) Upper respiratory rhinovirus infection
B) Allergic rhinitis
C) Hormonal rhinitis
D) Non allergic rhinitis with eosinophilia
E) Rhinitis medicamentosa

306) You are evaluating a 17-year-old girl with a 2 week history of rhinorrhea and nasal congestion that has kept her up at night. An over the counter nasal spray recommended by her friend, worked for 3-4 days but her symptoms have gotten a lot worse since then. She is otherwise a healthy straight A student with unremarkable growth and development. She is not sexually active, menstrual periods are regular and she is not taking oral contraceptive pills. On examination you note inflamed red turbinates that bleed easily. Nasal smear is negative. The most likely diagnosis would be:

A) Upper respiratory rhinovirus infection
B) Allergic rhinitis
C) Hormonal rhinitis
D) Non allergic rhinitis with eosinophilia
E) Rhinitis medicamentosa

307) Which of the following would be the most appropriate treatment for the patient described in the previous question?

A) Saline nose wash
B) Nasal corticosteroids
C) Nasal oxymetazoline
D) Oral oxymetazoline
E) Oral contraceptive pills

308) Appropriate treatment for the patient described in Question 306 could include each of the following *EXCEPT*:

A) Nasal saline irrigation
B) Nasal corticosteroids
C) Nasal azelastine
D) Nasal oxymetazoline
E) Nasal olopatadine

309) You are evaluating a 17 year old girl who presents with a several weeks history of clear rhinorrhea and intermittent sneezing. She is not complaining of itchy eyes or or nose. She is working this summer as a lifeguard at an indoor pool, as well as an assistant at her mother's hair salon. She is afebrile and otherwise asymptomatic. She is not sexually active, menstrual periods are regular and she is not taking oral contraceptive pills. On examination there is minimal swelling and no discoloration of the nasal turbinates. Her growth and development are unremarkable. A nasal smear reveals abundant eosinophils. She has not been taking any medications. The most likely diagnosis would be:

A) Upper respiratory rhinovirus infection
B) Allergic rhinitis
C) Hormonal rhinitis
D) Non allergic rhinitis with eosinophilia
E) Rhinitis medicamentosa

Adolescent Medicine and Gynecology

310) The parents of a 13-year-old girl are concerned about her pubertal development. On physical exam you note moderate breast development with glandular tissue beyond the areolae. However, you confirm that there is no secondary mounding of the nipples or areolae. Which of the following is the most appropriate sex maturity rating for breast development for this patient?

A) 1
B) 2
C) 3
D) 4
E) 5

311) A 12-year-old girl presents with intermittent white vaginal discharge over the past 2 to 3 months. She is Tanner stage 2 for breast and pubic hair staging and her physical exam is normal. Vaginal smear reveals 2 leukocytes/HPF as well as superficial vaginal cells. Which of the following is the MOST appropriate management?

A) 7 days of oral metronidazole
B) Testing for GC and Chlamydia
C) Immediate referral to child protective services
D) Reassurance that the discharge is normal
E) Topical clotrimazole for suspected Candidal infection

Questions

312) A 17-year-old football player has been fatigued since the conclusion of the football season one week ago. Prior to that time he had been doing well.

During the last game of the season he was hit in the left thigh during a tackle but he toughed it out and continued to play. On physical exam he still has pain and is walking with a limp. His white blood cell count is 10.0. His HCT is now 35, and at last year's physical examination he had an HCT of 42. His ESR is 6, his electrolytes are all within normal limits, his serum alkaline phosphatase is 200 and his lactic dehydrogenase is 225. The MOST likely diagnosis is:

A) Osteoid osteoma
B) Osteogenic sarcoma
C) Osteomyelitis
D) Deep thigh hematoma
E) Anabolic steroid use

313) You are asked to give a lecture to a group of high school coaches who want to know how to prevent "heat-related illnesses". Which of the following is the most appropriate recommendation?

A) Recommend they take 2 table salt tablets daily
B) Wear clothing that is loose fitting, light colored yet tasteful and not "Tutee Fruity"
C) Solar generated fans
D) Practice at night
E) Provide unrestricted access to fluids

314) Last month you evaluated an 18 year old male and prescribed 1 Gram single dose of azithromycin for a documented Chlamydia infection. He confirms that he has had only "one sexual partner" who he brings with him this time to be tested. He now presents with a one week history of urethritis with discharge confirmed on physical exam. Culture confirms that he once again has chlamydia urethritis. The most likely explanation for the recurrent infection is:

A) He has more than one sexual partner
B) Poor compliance with the prior treatment
C) Reinfection from his partner
D) He also has gonococcal urethritis
E) He needs a broader spectrum antibiotic

315) A rough formula for calculating the ideal body weight in females is:

A) 50 pounds for 50 inches in height plus 2 pounds for each additional inch
B) 75 pounds for 75 inches in height plus 5 pounds for each additional inch
C) 100 pounds for 60 inches in height plus 5 pounds for each additional inch
D) 125 pounds for every 72 inches of height plus 10 pounds for each additional inch
E) 125 pounds for every 72 inches of height plus 5 pounds for each additional inch

316) With regards to anorexia nervosa, each of the following represents an independent indication for hospital admission *EXCEPT*:

A) Heart rate greater than 100
B) Heart rate less than 40
C) Systolic blood pressure less than 90 mm Hg
D) Arrhythmia
E) Hypothermia

317) You are evaluating a 16 year old female presenting with dysfunctional uterine bleeding. Her menstrual cycles last 6 days and occur every 19 days. Her hemoglobin is 11 and her vital signs are stable. Each of the following would be appropriate treatment at this time *EXCEPT*:

A) Oral contraceptive pills
B) Serial hematocrits
C) Hospital admission for packed red cell transfusion
D) Iron supplements
E) Maintain a menstrual calendar

318) The gold standard for diagnosing genitourethral gonococcal infection is:

A) Culture grown on Thayer Martin medium
B) Culture grown on Chocolate Agar medium
C) Culture grown on Chocolate Martini medium
D) Nuclear acid amplification testing of patient obtained vaginal swab
E) Nucleic hybridization testing of urine samples in both male and female patients

Questions

319) You are evaluating a 17-year-old male who tests positive for *N. gonorrhea*. Which of the following is true regarding the management of his sexual partners?

   A) In states that allow it, prescribe appropriate treatment for all sexual partners within the past 6 months without an evaluation
   B) In states that allow it, prescribe appropriate treatment for all sexual partners within the past 60 days
   C) Recommend evaluation and treatment of all sexual partners he has had in his life
   D) Recommend evaluation and treatment of all sexual partners in the past 6 months
   E) Recommend evaluation and treatment of all sexual partners in the past 60 days

320) Which of the following is true regarding energy drinks in the teenage athlete?

   A) Energy drinks are effective at maintaining hydration
   B) Energy drinks contain guarana, which offsets the hypertensive effects of caffeine
   C) Ginseng, a common ingredient in energy drinks has been linked to breast tenderness and amenorrhea
   D) The daily-recommended allowance of caffeine is 150 mg daily
   E) Energy drinks are an excellent recommended source of taurine in teenagers who are ill

321) Teenagers and children drinking more than 300 mg of caffeine per day are at risk for the side effects of caffeine and caffeine withdrawal. Each of the following is among the effects of caffeine *EXCEPT*:

   A) Irritability
   B) Insomnia
   C) Drowsiness
   D) Osteoporosis
   E) Urinary retention

Sports Medicine

322) Which of the following conditions precludes participation in power lifting competition?

   A) Well controlled seizure disorder
   B) ADHD requiring stimulant medication
   C) Hypertension greater than 95th percentile for age
   D) Hypertension greater than 99th percentile for age
   E) Post exertional syncope

323) Which of the following is consistent with recommendations for weight control in young athletes of the American Academy of Pediatrics?

   A) A body fat content of 15% is considered to be very high for the female teen athlete
   B) A body fat content of 10% is considered to be high for the male teen athlete
   C) Standard body mass index to assess weight in relation to height is appropriate regardless of muscle mass
   D) Long distance runners needing to lose weight should do so gradually under close medical supervision
   E) Cyclic weight loss during the season coupled with weight gain in the off season is appropriate during growth spurts

324) Each of the following is true regarding children wishing to do strength training prior to puberty *EXCEPT*:

   A) Most injuries are due to mishandling of weights
   B) Supervision is critical to appropriate strength training
   C) Documentation of normotension is important
   D) Proper form can only be practiced with heavy weights
   E) Well-designed resistance training programs can be safe and beneficial in athletes as young as 6

Questions

325) Which of the following is true regarding exercise in children?

A) Physical activity in childhood is associated with decreased risk for coronary heart disease in adulthood
B) Lower socioeconomic status has been correlated with higher rates of participation in sports
C) 2/3 of high school students meet the CDC recommendation for 60 minutes of moderate to vigorous exercise each day
D) Children are more likely to engage in organized sports when parents are supportive of this
E) There is no correlation between physical activity in childhood and physical activity later in adulthood

326) You are seeing a 17 year old boy for knee pain that has been getting worse over the past week. He plays football and first felt the pain after he was tackled in practice last week. He tried to continue playing but has not been able to participate fully due to pain on the inside of his knee. He does not recall any locking or popping sensation although he is limping and guarding his knee; there is no effusion or erythema noted. The patella moves appropriately with flexion and extension. Pain is limited to the medial aspect of the knee with valgus stress. There is no swelling or effusion noted. There is no locking while walking up and down stairs. The most likely diagnosis would be:

A) Medial meniscus tear
B) Lateral meniscus tear
C) Medial collateral ligament strain
D) Lateral collateral ligament strain
E) Anterior cruciate ligament tear

Substance Abuse

327) Which one of the following statements with regards to amphetamines and methamphetamines is *TRUE*?

A) The N-methyl group on methamphetamine results in decreased peripheral side effects
B) Amphetamines work by decreasing presynaptic uptake
C) D-form and L-form are equal pharmacokinetically
D) Phentolamine and nifedipine are used in acute overdose situations
E) Haloperidol is used to treat the aggression/agitation that often accompanies amphetamine abuse

328) You are working as a camp doctor primarily to relax and get free tuition for your kid. You are reeling in a small mouth bass, when you are awoken by the hum of an approaching panic stricken crowd. Apparently it is 9AM and you were only dreaming about fishing.

They bring in a 12 year old boy believed to be drunk. He was found in the woods near his bunk, laughing, ataxic, and slurring his words. Fortunately you have a drug test which is negative for alcohol, Cannibis and all drugs on the panel.

You observe the boy for an hour and the symptoms quickly resolve over 30 minutes.

The most likely diagnosis explanation for the clinical presentation would be:

A) Lab error
B) Glue inhalation
C) Malingering behavior
D) Poison mushroom ingestion
E) Poppy Seed toxicity

329) Sudden death from cocaine toxicity would most likely be due to

A) Trauma secondary to inappropriate behavior
B) Cardiac arrhythmias
C) Barotrauma following Valsalva maneuver to increase inhalation
D) Cerebral vascular accident secondary to hypertension
E) Bilateral pneumothoraces

330) You are evaluating a sleepy teenager in the emergency room. Pupils are equal and normal sized but react sluggishly to light. The conjunctiva are not injected.

Which of the following substances could account for these clinical findings?

A) Alprazolam
B) Amphetamine
C) Phencyclidine
D) Heroin
E) Marijuana

331) You are evaluating a teenager who, while playing football, suddenly collapses on the field. You evaluate him and he is disoriented to time and place and is tachycardic, tachypneic and has a recorded fever of 104.5. His pupils are equal, reactive and normal size.

Which of the following would be most appropriate in treating this patient once his airway and breathing have been established?

A) Provide him with a cool glass of water
B) Rapid cooling to 101.8F but no lower
C) Rapid cooling to 98.6
D) Naloxone
E) IV dextrose rapid infusion

332) We live in a world of e-scribing of prescriptions; email instead of snail mail, EMR instead of plain medical records but efforts to E-liminate cigarette smoking have been blunted by the increased popularity of electronic or E-cigarettes. Which of the following is true regarding electronic cigarettes?

A) There is conclusive evidence that electronic cigarettes are effective for smoking cessation
B) The vapor exhaled by users may contain nicotine
C) Flavoring is now banned by the FDA making them less attractive to children
D) The vaporization technique and nicotine content is closely regulated
E) Advertising is limited and controlled

Disorders of Cognition, Language and Learning

333) At what age is a toddler normally 75% understandable to a stranger?

   A) 24 months
   B) 36 months
   C) 18 months
   D) 18 years
   E) Presidential candidate

334) Identifying children with developmental delays, is best achieved by:

   A) EEG monitoring while watching the auditions for American Idol
   B) Standardized developmental screening at every well child visit
   C) Asking parents if their child is developing normally
   D) Screening all children for vision and hearing
   E) Screening for inborn errors of metabolism at birth

335) A 14 year old male with intellectual disability presents with a past medical history that is unremarkable. The family history is essentially positive for a couple of uncles who, according to the mother, "are 5 beers short of a 6-pack" and according to the father, "were one top short of the 4 tops".

   On physical exam you note a long face that would rival Richard Belzer on Law and Order, large ears and macroorchidism. This disorder would BEST be diagnosed with which study?

   A) Head CT
   B) Head MRI
   C) Karyotype
   D) EEG
   E) DNA testing

Behavior and Mental Health

336) In addition to cognitive behavioral psychotherapy, each of the following could be considered in a 16 year old suffering from a binge-eating disorder, <u>EXCEPT</u>:

   A) Imipramine
   B) Topiramate
   C) Lisdexamfetamine
   D) Sertraline
   E) Citalopram

337) You are evaluating a previously well 15 year old boy. His parents are concerned because he has reached "Jeb Bush levels of low energy".[7] He Is going to sleep earlier and getting up later, often missing the school bus. His teachers report that he is having a difficult time concentrating in class. Previously he was an enthusiastic participant on the varsity basketball team, but now has been skipping practice and weighs 175 pounds, up from 150 three months ago . He denies any drug or alcohol use, and the parents do not suspect he is using drugs.

   Each of the following would be appropriate immediate steps in the diagnosis and management of this patient except:

   A) Complete Blood Count
   B) Thyroid studies
   C) Assess his safety and risk for harm to himself or others
   D) Counsel him and schedule a followup visit in 3 months
   E) Interview parents and patient separately regarding situation

---

[7] Parents neither confirm nor deny that they were a supporter of Donald Trump when asked. They were just trying to add some levity to a dire situation.

338) You are seeing a 10 year old boy during his routine physical examination in October. In the past, he had exhibited impulsivity and inattention both at home and at school. 2 years ago, he was started on a course of methylphenidate, and there has been moderate improvement in his ability to sustain attention at school and decreased impulsivity at home. However, this year his teachers have reported his being more disruptive at school. He has been disrespectful to teachers and other staff at school. He often mocks and makes fun of the teachers behind their backs and seems disinterested in learning math and reading. At home he has not exhibited such behaviors except when pushed to do his homework or when help is offered at home with his school work. Which of the following would be the most appropriate next step?

A) Increase the dose of methylphenidate
B) Switch to atomoxetine
C) Behavioral modification to extinguish the behavior
D) Psychoeducational evaluation
E) Switch reading and math teachers

339) Which of the following would be the most appropriate first step in managing a 6 year old exhibiting signs of oppositional –defiance ?

A) Individual play therapy sessions with a trained counselor
B) Ask the child to reflect on how his behavior impacts everyone else
C) Remind the child that he is difficult and show how him that other children are better behaved
D) Implement behavioral management modification steps worked out with a child behavioral specialist
E) Prescribe lisdexamfetamine

340) Which of the following is true regarding the diagnosis and treatment of Attention Deficit with Hyperactivity (ADHD) in children?

A) A history of inattention and impulsivity at school is sufficient to establish the diagnosis
B) A diagnostic and therapeutic trial of stimulant medication is the recommended initial step
C) Learning disabilities are rarely seen in children after they have been treated successfully with stimulant medications
D) Early cognitive milestones in the normal range are rarely reported in children with ADHD
E) Hyperactivity and impulsive behavior must be observed in at least 2 settings

Psychosocial

341) Which subgroup of teenagers is at the highest risk for suicide?

A) Drug users
B) Children of divorce
C) Those dealing with sexual identity issues
D) Teens on ADHD medication
E) Those with chronic medical conditions

342) Children with *mild* intellectual disability are more likely to:

A) Show marked delays in psychomotor skills in the first year of life
B) Have delayed speech and language abilities in the toddler years
C) Have a history of perinatal problems
D) Be diagnosed at school entry
E) Have a physical deformity

343) While autism is largely understood to be an idiopathic disorder, it has been associated with each of the following conditions *EXCEPT*:

A) Trisomy 21
B) Untreated phenylketonuria
C) Tuberous sclerosis
D) Fragile X syndrome
E) Anoxia during birth

344) Regarding dyslexia, each of the following statements is true *EXCEPT*:

A) It is frequently discovered in the fourth grade
B) It can go undetected into adulthood
C) It is an uncommon language disorder
D) There is evidence of a possible anatomical basis for the disorder
E) It tends to run in families

345) You are seeing a 3-year-old for a routine physical examination. The history and physical are unremarkable. Development and interactions are normal for age except for marked delay in speech. This is MOST suggestive of:

A) Infantile autism
B) Tongue-tie
C) Hearing loss
D) Bilingual household
E) Intellectual disability

346) Our next contestant on "Name That Age" is an infant who is able to babble and transfer a cube from one hand to another, yet drops one cube when handed another. He can crawl but does so by dragging his belly across the floor like a marine sneaking into enemy territory. These developmental milestones are MOST consistent with which age?

A) 5 months
B) 7 months
C) 9 months
D) 11 months
E) 18 years

347) The next contestant on Name That Age lifts his head and chest while lying down, coos, visually follows his mother around the room, and has a "primitive grasp" but cannot yet hold his rattle. The MOST likely age is:

A) 1 month
B) 2 months
C) 4 months
D) 6 months
E) 9 months

Questions

348) A couple who has recently adopted a newborn infant is here for the 2-week visit. They would like to know if and when the child should be told he was adopted. The BEST time to tell children of their adoption would be:

   A) When they bring it up themselves
   B) If there are other siblings, it is best to avoid the topic
   C) The age of 10, when they are mature enough to handle the information
   D) When their verbal development allows for comprehension; around the age of 3 or 4 years
   E) Never!

349) A mother of a child in your practice cannot deny that her child is suffering from ADHD. However, she was referred to you because you are "open-minded" when it comes to treatment, and she wants to use "natural remedies" rather than the medications she has heard about that "turn kids into zombies" so lazy teachers do not have to do their jobs. Based on the latest findings your best approach would be to:

   A) Discuss the benefits of Kava Kava
   B) Review the benefits of a trial of Valerian root and reinforcement of organizational skills and behavior
   C) Review the child's diet for any preservatives, sugars, and dyes known to trigger ADHD, and speak with the teacher about seating arrangements
   D) Discuss the benefits of a combination of herbs and supplements, including Kava Kava, Valerian root, Ginkgo biloba, and fish oil
   E) Reassure her, evaluate her fears, and review what is known about methylphenidate and other medications to treat ADHD. Also discuss other non-medication methods to manage the condition, like behavior management

350) The parents of a 6-month-old girl consult you because the infant has been crying uncontrollably for the past 2 hours. Physical examination reveals an incarcerated inguinal hernia that you are able to reduce with some difficulty. You recommend that the hernia be repaired soon and explain the risk of recurrence of incarceration as well as the benefits and risks of surgery. The parents request that the surgery be delayed until the girl is at least one year of age. Of the following, your next step should be to:

   A) Explore the parent's reasons for wishing to delay the surgery
   B) Obtain a court order to proceed with surgery
   C) Let the parents know if they ignore an incarcerated hernia they will be incarcerated
   D) Refer the parents to another physician
   E) Tell the parents that the risks of surgery are minimal

351) The parents of a 24-month-old boy are concerned because he displays ritualistic behavior. He has tantrums if he is interrupted, and he appears withdrawn. Which of the following is most likely to be associated with this child's problem?

A) Appropriate gesturing to indicate needs
B) Stranger anxiety
C) Abnormal language development
D) Hearing deficit
E) Maintenance of sustained eye contact

352) The parent of an 18-month-old girl consults you regarding the girl's language development. The girl has a 12-word vocabulary and uses a considerable amount of jargon, but she does not use any two-word phrases. Of the following, the best course of action at this time would be to:

A) Refer the girl for tympanometry
B) Refer the girl for brain stem evoked audiometry
C) Refer the girl to a speech pathologist
D) Refer the girl for a complete developmental evaluation
E) Assure the parent that language development is normal

353) You are giving a talk to a group of residents on the topic of sexual identity in teens. Which of the following would be true?

A) Sexual orientation and gender identity are synonymous
B) Sexual orientation is based solely on genetic predisposition
C) Homosexual teenagers are less likely to drop out of high school than their heterosexual peers
D) Sexual behavior and activity is a choice
E) Parents should be told that their children are free to choose their sexual orientation

354) A single mother brings her 7 year old daughter to be evaluated because she has found her in front of the television rubbing and touching her genitals on more than one occasion. The girl lives with mom but spends every other weekend at dad's.

Which of the following additional behaviors would raise concern?

A) The girl's interest in wearing men's clothing
B) Vaginal discharge
C) Vaginal irritation
D) Imitation of adult sexual acts
E) Reluctance to undress in front of the mother

355) What would be the appropriate approach to a family with a child with a chronic, progressively debilitating illness that has kept the details away from him?

A) Continue to keep the information a secret until it is too obvious to hide
B) Encourage them to explain the illness in terms developmentally appropriate for age
C) Note that if they don't tell the child, you will
D) Note that denying information from the child is akin to neglect requiring you to report them to the authorities
E) Suggest the child's teacher break the news to him

356) Each of the following is true regarding separation anxiety disorder *EXCEPT*:

A) It is characterized by periods of exacerbation and remission
B) It occurs primarily in males
C) Symptoms can continue into adulthood
D) Peak onset is middle childhood
E) These children often have other psychiatric disorders

357) Resumption of school attendance after a time away from school is best performed by:

A) Having the parent stay in school for gradually decreased periods of time
B) Have the child initially attend on alternate days
C) A combination of home and school tutoring on alternating weeks
D) Immediate return without parent
E) Immediate return with liberal use of pharmacological agents

Critical Care

358) It is 2 AM in the PICU. It is your 5th night on call in 4 days. You need to start a child on a ventilator, and you need to quickly calculate the tidal volume for this 15kg child. The correct tidal volume is closest to:

   A) 1500 ml
   B) 150 ml
   C) 100 ml
   D) 60 ml
   E) 35 ml
   F) 6 trillion ml

359) This month you are working in the PICU and you are successfully managing a case of botulism poisoning. You are there catching up on your dictation, noting the steady drone of the mom clicking on her laptop when she stops, your eyes meet and she says, "So Doc, what exactly is the mechanism of action of botulism toxin?"

   You've done your homework and correctly answer:

   A) It increases reuptake of acetylcholine at the presynaptic neuron
   B) It blocks the mom's laptop from "googling" botulism toxin
   C) It destroys the postsynaptic membrane
   D) It blocks release of acetylcholine from the presynaptic neuron
   E) It blocks the reuptake of acetylcholine

360) You arrive just as lifeguards are pulling out a toddler who is limp, unconscious, and making minimal respiratory efforts. The best immediate intervention would be:

   A) The Heimlich maneuver to clear the airway of water
   B) Turn the child on the prone position and administer 3 back blows
   C) Place the child on his back and lift his left leg up and down pumping aspirated water out of his mouth, like in Tom and Jerry and other cartoons
   D) Initiate BLS including rescue breathing and chest compressions if indicated
   E) Immobilize cervical spine and call 911

361) Which of the following is the *diagnostic triad* of Acute Respiratory Distress Syndrome (ARDS)?

A) Cardiogenic pulmonary edema, impaired oxygenation, bilateral pulmonary infiltrates
B) Noncardiogenic pulmonary edema, impaired oxygenation, bilateral pulmonary infiltrates
C) Renal failure, impaired oxygenation, unilateral pulmonary infiltrates
D) Renal failure, impaired oxygenation, bilateral pulmonary infiltrates
E) Noncardiogenic pulmonary edema, acidosis, bilateral pulmonary infiltrates

Emergency Medicine

362) Each of the following may be administered via an endotracheal tube *EXCEPT*:

   A) Lidocaine
   B) Epinephrine
   C) Sodium bicarbonate
   D) Atropine
   E) Naloxone HCl

363) You are following an 8 month old in the ER who initially presented with moderate respiratory distress. He has responded well to a series of albuterol treatments. Your decision to discharge him from the ER vs. admit him for additional treatment should take into account all of the following *EXCEPT*:

   A) Parental reliability
   B) Paramyxovirus as the underlying cause
   C) Oral intake and hydration status
   D) Use of racemic epinephrine while in the ER
   E) Resolution of the symptoms after a period of observation

364) You are called to the ER where a mom and a 3 month old are waiting for you. Mom is in a custody battle in a nasty divorce[8] and she points to a red raised spot on the child's abdomen which may have been present at birth but "it is definitely worse after spending a week with his father". "Not only that," adds the grandmother as she walks in shaking off her umbrella on the code tray and your clogs, "look at the black and blue marks on his lower back and the one on his ankles." You notice that the black and blue marks are all the same color with no variation, and the raised red pattern is also not tender. You inform the mother, grandmother (grandfather who was staring at the wall the whole time) that:

A) You will document this clear case of paternal child abuse and cooperate with their attorney free of charge if necessary
B) The red rash is a strawberry hemangioma that will naturally get worse before it gets better, and the black and blue marks are Mongolian spots that they probably did not notice earlier. There is no abuse suspected
C) You will call Child Protective Services to document this and have them interview the mother to make sure it wasn't she who inflicted the damage and is only trying to cover herself
D) You join the grandfather and comment on the color of the wall
E) You will admit the child for further testing

365) Each of the following is often used in the treatment of acute methamphetamine intoxication *EXCEPT*:

A) Phentolamine
B) Nifedipine
C) Beta blockers
D) IV normal saline
E) Lorazepam

366) A 5-year-old child is intubated and mechanically ventilated following respiratory arrest secondary to septic shock. Twenty-four hours later, his HR is 45 and BP is 135/105 mm Hg. The most urgently required intervention at this time would be:

A) 12-lead EKG
B) Vasodilators IV
C) Insertion of a central venous catheter
D) Lumbar puncture
E) Hyperventilation

---

8 Is there any other kind?

367) A 16 year-old girl is brought to the ED. She is comatose and unresponsive to verbal or painful stimuli. You start a normal saline bolus and secure her airway. Temperature is 35.8 C, with a heart rate of 65, respiratory rate of 6, and BP of 84/56. Muscle tone is flaccid. Pupils are equal but constricted. Blood glucose concentration is 225 mg/dL. The MOST appropriate next step would be to administer:

A) Naloxone
B) Physostigmine
C) Atropine
D) Epinephrine
E) Glucose

368) The *most* serious consequence of glue sniffing is:

A) Chronic rhinitis
B) Ataxia
C) Cardiac arrhythmia
D) Hallucinations
E) Lead encephalopathy
F) Glueing your nostrils together :)

369) A 16-year-old boy is diagnosed with acute appendicitis and emergency surgery is necessary. The patient is a severe persistent asthmatic on chronic oral steroids.

The MOST appropriate management in anticipation of surgery would be:

A) Perform an ACTH stimulation test
B) Measure serum cortisol concentration
C) Measure serum glucose concentration
D) Begin high-dose inhaled corticosteroid therapy
E) Administer perioperative corticosteroids IV

Questions

370) Each of the following would be appropriate steps in managing hypokalemia *EXCEPT*:

A) Cardiorespiratory monitoring
B) Administration of potassium
C) Administration of insulin and glucose
D) IV fluids
E) Monitoring of acid – base balance

371) A 14-year-old has a two-day history of progressively worsening vomiting, chills and RUQ abdominal pain. Her WBC is 22,000. Urine Cx grows >100,000 colonies of *E. coli*/mL of urine. Which of the following is the MOST likely diagnosis?

A) Renal stones
B) Cystitis
C) Cholecystitis
D) Acute pyelonephritis
E) Gallstones

372) A 13-year-old boy who fell while skateboarding was unconscious for 5-7 minutes. He does not recall what happened immediately after he fell and is not complaining of a headache. He has vomited twice since the fall.

On physical exam, he is alert and oriented with a Glasgow Coma Scale score of 14. There is no blood behind his tympanic membrane and no nasal discharge. His neurological examination is normal as is the remainder of the physical exam. The MOST appropriate next step in managing this patient would be:

A) X-ray of the skull
B) Urinalysis
C) Abdominal ultrasound
D) CT scan of the head
E) Overnight observation; additional studies pending clinical status

373) A 17-year-old boy is brought to the ED by ambulance. He was found at home more disoriented and confused than usual.[9] He is ataxic with increased deep tendon reflexes, muscle rigidity, increased salivation, and nystagmus. He is also exhibiting catatonic behavior. His BP is 170/100. Which of the following is the MOST likely diagnosis?

  A) Phencyclidine intoxication
  B) LSD intoxication
  C) Opiate intoxication
  D) Hyperventilation syndrome
  E) Hysteria

374) A 13-year-old is brought to the ED directly from school after being "jumped" by several classmates. In addition to a sore arm and a hematoma on his forehead, he complains that his nose hurts and that he is having difficulty breathing. He is tender of the bridge of his nose and there is marked swelling of the nasal septum, resulting in virtual occlusion of both nares. The *most appropriate* next step would be:

  A) Head CT
  B) X-ray of the nasal bones and zygomatic arch
  C) Play the theme from new release of Rocky
  D) Have him seen by ENT within one week once swelling has subsided
  E) Evaluation by ENT as soon as possible

375) A 4-1/2-year-old lethargic child is brought to you from the triage area. Up until now, the child's medical history had been unremarkable. The child's mother is being treated for depression. Each of the following would be appropriate measures <u>EXCEPT</u>:

  A) 12-lead EKG
  B) Oxygen saturation monitor
  C) Syrup of ipecac
  D) Activated charcoal
  E) Endotracheal intubation

---

9 Even more than the disorientation and confusion that is baseline for the average teenager.

Questions

376) Which of the following findings could have a likely explanation OTHER THAN child abuse?

   A) 6-month-old presenting with fussiness, a tender leg, and a metaphyseal fracture of the proximal tibia
   B) A very active 2-year-old with bruising on the shin and evidence of multiple healed fractures secondary to falling
   C) 3-year-old with rib fractures and who is taking ice skating lessons
   D) 5-year-old with a skull fracture first noted in the morning by the parents
   E) 3-month-old with soft tissue swelling of the face and jaw and evidence of cortical thickening of the long and flat bones

377) Deferoxamine is administered IV to a child who ingested an unknown amount of ferrous sulfate. Shortly after administration, the urine has a pink color. The physiological explanation for this is that:

   A) Free serum iron has been chelated with deferoxamine and excreted in the urine
   B) Insufficient iron was ingested to chelate all the deferoxamine, which is then excreted in the urine
   C) Unbound serum transferrin has been chelated with deferoxamine and excreted in the urine
   D) Hemoglobin-iron has been chelated with deferoxamine, causing hemolysis and hemoglobinuria
   E) The serum iron concentration exceeds the chelating capacity of deferoxamine, allowing free iron excretion in the urine

378) The most common form of child abuse is:

   A) Emotional deprivation
   B) Verbal abuse
   C) Physical abuse
   D) Sexual abuse
   E) Neglect

379) A mother reports by telephone that her 4-year-old daughter fell from a wagon and hit her head on the sidewalk. The girl was unresponsive for one minute. She has vomited twice and is now sleepy but easily aroused. You would most *appropriately* advise the mother to:

   A) Keep the child quiet, administer aspirin for headache, and let her continue to sleep
   B) Examine the child every hour for pupillary size and reactivity, and bring her to the ER if either pupil enlarges or reacts poorly
   C) Bring the child to the hospital for careful clinical evaluation
   D) Take the child to the hospital for x-ray study of the skull
   E) Administer small doses of phenobarbital at home for the next 48 hours

380) Each of the following is true regarding the use of ketamine for conscious sedation *EXCEPT*:

   A) It produces sensory blockade
   B) It can trigger "emergence hallucinations"
   C) It decreases secretions
   D) It is useful for short painful procedures
   E) It is often used in conjunction with midazolam

381) Midazolam has each of the following characteristics *EXCEPT*:

   A) Analgesic
   B) Amnesic
   C) Anxiolytic
   D) Sedating
   E) Enigmatic

Questions

382) An afebrile 9 month old is brought to the emergency department with intermittent episodes of crampy abdominal pain and bilious vomiting. On physical exam you note right lower quadrant tenderness. In between episodes of pain, the patient is reported to be lethargic. You note a "coiled spring" appearance on radiography.

The most likely diagnosis would be:

A) Your hallucinating the coiled spring out of a desire to pop a champagne bottle and retire
B) Swallowed foreign body
C) Hirschprung's disease
D) Intussusception
E) Duodenal atresia

383) A 15 year old presents with a headache, pain with swallowing. Although he is afebrile now, he notes that he felt very hot earlier in the day before taking ibuprofen. He has raised rough, fine bumps on his trunk and lower abdomen that blanch easily. The most appropriate next step in this patient would be:

A) CBC , Blood culture and immediate IV Ceftriaxone
B) Abdominal ultrasound
C) Abdominal CT with IV and PO contrast
D) Rapid Strep and throat culture
E) Urineanalysis

384) A 15 year old presents with headache, weakness and urinary frequency. He has lost weight recently and has been dinking a lot of water lately while training for football season. His coach has been upset because his usual effort is not there. In addition the coach notes the smell of acetone when the patient is doing drills and suspects he is sniffing glue.

Which of the following would be the most appropriate next step in diagnosing the cause of this presentation?

A) CBC and Blood culture
B) Urine drug screen
C) Abdominal ultrasound
D) Abdominal CT scan with PO and IV contrast
E) Urineanalysis

Pharmacology and Pain Management

385) A teenager taking oral contraceptive pills should be concerned regarding its efficacy when taking which of the following herbal remedies?

   A) Valerian Root
   B) Echinacea
   C) Ginseng
   D) Mooderall
   E) St. John's Wort

386) Which of the following herbal remedies is contraindicated in patients taking immunosuppressant medications?

   A) Echinacea
   B) Ginseng
   C) Sing Sing
   D) St. John's Wort
   E) Valerian Root

387) Which of the following herbal remedies should type 2 diabetics taking oral hypoglycemic medications be concerned about?

   A) Echinacea
   B) Ginseng
   C) Valerian Root
   D) St. John's Wort
   E) Peppermint tea

Questions

388) You are participating in a clinical trial. In fact, it is the "Clinical Trial of the Century" on Judge Joe Brown so you'd better get this question right or else Jimmy Kimmel will be reviewing your pharmacological credentials on his live TV show. The medication is given twice a day and it reaches a steady state after 5 days. The half life of the drug is closest to:

   A) 12 hours
   B) 24 hours
   C) 36 hours
   D) 72 hours
   E) Who cares?

389) Each of the following conditions can alter the serum level and, therefore, the bioavailability and toxicity of a variety of medications *EXCEPT*:

   A) Severe burns
   B) Liver disease
   C) Nephrotic syndrome
   D) Hypertension
   E) Juvenile polyps

Research and Statistics

390) Which of the following is true regarding prospective cohort studies?

A) Time sequence cannot be established
B) It is impossible to infer causality
C) There are never losses to followup
D) It is an excellent method to study whether exposure precedes the outcome being studied
E) A small cohort is preferred for studying rare outcomes

391) Which of the following is true regarding a systematic review of literature?

A) Systematic review of literature cannot be valid without meta-analysis
B) Systematic review of literature is a random process but valid as long as it is thorough
C) All identified studies must be included in the review
D) Publication bias often results in the exclusion of studies that demonstrate statistically relevant positive results.
E) The Cochrane library is an independent compilations of systematic reviews of medical topics

392) Which of the following is true regarding meta-analysis?

A) Summary statistics give equal weight to all studies regardless of the number of subjects
B) Summary statistics give more weight to studies with fewer subjects
C) Summary statistics give more weight to studies with more subjects
D) Homogeneity and heterogeneity are no longer factors in today's politically correct approach to research analysis
E) Unpublished statistically relevant negative studies should not be factored into meta-analysis

393) Which of the following is true regarding case control studies?

A) It is used for studying diagnostic tests
B) It requires more subjects than a cohort study
C) It is effective in studying rare diseases with long latency periods
D) You can only study the impact of 1 risk factor
E) It is very time consuming

394) Each of the following is true regarding randomized controlled trial studies *EXCEPT*:

A) Results can be analyzed with established statistical tools
B) Causation can easily be established
C) Is a costly method of study
D) It is at risk for volunteer bias
E) Confounding variables can diminish the validity of the findings

Ethics for Primary Care Physicians

395) Which of the following is true regarding transgender youth?

   A) Psychiatric comorbidity is very uncommon in transgender youth
   B) Reparative psychotherapy should be implemented before confirming a diagnosis of gender dysphoria
   C) Intervention for gender dysphoria prior to adulthood is limited to counseling and medical workup
   D) Pubertal suppression through gonadotropin-releasing hormone (GnRH) analogs allows for a smoother social and physical transition to the gender role congruent with gender identity
   E) The role of the pediatrician is to explore gender dysphoria only when approached by the child or the family

396) Which of the following is true regarding children serving as living solid organ or stem cell donors?

   A) Purposeful conception of additional children in the hopes of finding an ideal stem cell match is never appropriate
   B) Meaningful assent is always factored in regardless of age
   C) Meaningful assent is never factored in regardless of age
   D) Siblings with cognitive disabilities are often the first choice among siblings for organ donation
   E) Regarding solid organ donation, assent without coercion must be established by an independent advocacy team

397) You are managing a patient who has been diagnosed with osteogenic carcinoma. The parents would like a 3 month trial of bioelectromagnetic therapy before starting recommended chemotherapy and radiation therapy. Which of the following would be the most appropriate management in this situation:

   A) Implement a trial of bioelectromagnetic therapy as long as it is coupled with biofield therapy
   B) Shake your head and say fugghedeboutit !
   C) Refuse to implement bioelectromagnetic therapy on the grounds that it is a violation of beneficence
   D) Patient autonomy mandates that you comply with the parents wishes
   E) Review any potential adverse effects of the bioelectromagnetic therapy and discuss using it alongside traditional evidence based management

Questions

398) A family has moved to your area and is opposed to immunizing the children. Each of the following would be appropriate information in counseling this family *EXCEPT*:

   A) The risk for encephalopathy due the measles vaccine is 1 in a million
   B) The risk for encephalopathy from measles is 1 in a thousand
   C) Vaccines in general are low risk / high benefit
   D) The latest vaccines are 100% effective
   E) The decision can impact the wellbeing of other children in the community

399) You have been contacted by a local attorney to provide expert testimony in court. Each of the following is an appropriate ethical guideline regarding expert testimony and consultation in legal proceedings *EXCEPT*:

   A) Transcripts of court testimony are exempt from peer review
   B) It is ethical for pediatricians to testify in court as experts when they are mandated to appear
   C) It is ethical for pediatricians to testify in court as experts even if they are not mandated to do so
   D) It is reasonable to receive appropriate compensation as an expert witness in the same state where the physician is licensed and practices
   E) Compensation for court appearance should never be contingent on the outcome of the case

Patient Safety and Quality Improvement

400) Which of the following best describes a *sentinel* event ?

A) Unanticipated death or injury as a result of a medical error
B) Unanticipated death or injury as a result of medical care
C) An error that is noted before it impacts the patient
D) An error performed by a security guard
E) A medical error that is due to faulty handwriting

401) Which of the following is the definition of a *medical error*?

A) Unanticipated death or injury as a result of medical care
B) An error that is noted before it impacts the patient
C) A preventable adverse effect of care that is evident or harmful to the patient
D) A failure to complete a planned action as intended, or the use of a wrong plan to achieve an aim
E) An adverse event that is due to a medication error

402) Each of the following is true regarding *near miss events* <u>EXCEPT</u>:

A) A near miss event can be intercepted
B) A near miss event can occur without being intercepted
C) A non-intercepted near miss event always results in harm to the patient
D) A near miss event can be a result of incorrect keyboard entry into an EMR
E) Near miss events are caused by medical error

403) Each of the following is true regarding adverse events <u>EXCEPT</u>:

A) Most medical errors are not adverse events
B) An adverse event may be caused either by medical management *or by* the underlying disease or condition of the patient
C) An adverse drug event (ADE) is an adverse event that is due an administered medication
D) All adverse events result in harm to the patient
E) There are two types of adverse events: preventable and non-preventable.

Questions

404) Which of the following is true regarding medical errors?

A) Medical errors always lead to harm to the patient
B) All medical errors should be tracked and reviewed
C) Only medical errors causing harm to the patient should be tracked
D) All sentinel events are due to medical error
E) All adverse drug events are preventable

Answers

Answers

Nutrition

1) C) Breast milk is known to contain IgA, immunomodulating agents to enhance the breast-feeding infant's own immune system, anti-inflammatory agents, and anti-microbial agents.

However choice C, IgG would be incorrect since IgG is *not* present in breast milk.

2)
1) (B)
2) (E)
3) (A)
4) (D)
5) (C)

Retinol (Vitamin A) deficiency is the leading cause of blindness worldwide.

Tocopherol (Vitamin E) deficiency is associated with hemolytic anemia.

Deficiency of phylloquinone, or vitamin K is associated with hemorrhagic disease of the newborn.

Thiamine (Vitamin B1) deficiency is associated with peripheral paralysis and muscle weakness.

Riboflavin (Vitamin B2) deficiency is associated with angular stomatitis and seborrheic dermatitis.

3)
1) (C)
2) (B)
3) (A)

Tocopherol which is also known as vitamin E can result in liver toxicity.

Niacin also known as vitamin B_3 can result in vasodilation if taken in toxic doses.

Ascorbic acid or vitamin C taken in excessive dosages can lead to nephrocalcinosis.

4) D) Calciferol is another name for vitamin D. **Vitamin D deficiency** can result in high serum phosphatase levels, infantile tetany, poor growth and osteomalacia.

Calciferol regulates the absorption and deposition of calcium and phosphorus. High serum phosphatase levels can appear prior to the bone deformities seen with rickets.

However calciferol or vitamin D deficiency does not result in pharyngeal ulcers.

5) B) Niacin (Vitamin B_3) deficiency can result in pellagra, which manifests as GI distress, dementia, and skin manifestations, including rash.

Xerophthalmia is associated with vitamin A (retinol) deficiency, not niacin deficiency.

6) D) The clinical description is of scurvy which is seen in infants fed evaporated milk without supplementation. The irritability, generalized tenderness (the explanation for the child being irritable and not wanting to be touched), petechiae, gum swelling are all consistent with vitamin C (ascorbic acid) deficiency.

The x-ray findings, thinning of the cortices, ground glass appearance of the bones and calcified cartilage at the metaphysis are also consistent with scurvy.

The most appropriate treatment would be ascorbic acid supplementation.

7) D) Joint aches, headache and lethargy are all consistent with retinol or vitamin A toxicity. The increased opening pressure on LP would be consistent with this diagnosis and the absence of white blood cells in an atraumatic tap (absence of red blood cells) would rule out aseptic meningitis.

There is nothing in the history to suggest trauma or migraine headaches. Retinol deficiency would not present with these symptoms.

Answers

8) **A)** The skin color, prematurity and exclusive breast feeding places this child at risk for vitamin D deficiency and the clinical picture of rickets.

There is nothing to suggest a diagnosis of vitamin, E, D or A deficiency. Likewise there is nothing to suggest a diagnosis of iron deficiency or cystic fibrosis.

9) **E)** Despite the urban medical myth of the BRATT diet, the appropriate treatment if tolerated is oral rehydration and a regular diet to assure that the child is getting adequate nutrition.

The only restriction would be fluids containing a high concentration of sugar.

10) **D)** If you remember the adage "if the gut works use it" this is an easy question. The presence of absence of air fluid levels will be critical in knowing if the gut isn't working.

Enteral feeding is always preferred especially since it is known to actually decrease inflammation and stimulate the production of digestive enzymes. Parenteral feedings should be avoided since it lacks these advantages, plus there is the added risk of line infection and other complications.

11) **D)** Home prepared foods do not decrease the risk of food allergies. Standard bottled vegetables may contain more sugar and salt than an infant can tolerate so home prepared vegetables are preferred. Honey should never be given to an infant during the first year of life.

Home prepared products should be pureed and *can be frozen and used later.*

12) **D)** Breastfeeding like most gifts benefits the giver and the receiver. Mothers who breastfeed are at lower risk for breast as well as ovarian cancer, type 2 diabetes and postpartum depression.

There is an *increased* rate of weight loss in the immediate post-partum period. In other words weight is lost more quickly.

Preventive Pediatrics

13) D) Children older than 2-1/2 need to receive no more than 35% of their caloric intake from fat. All the other choices are incorrect. Screening should be started at 2 not 1. If family history alone were used as a parameter in choosing whom to screen, many children with hypercholesterolemia would be missed. Also, hypercholesteremia can have many causes such as nephrotic syndrome and hypothyroidism. It is a low HDL, which is a worrisome sign in both children and adults. The opposite is true with LDL, that is, a low LDL is a good sign and a high LDL is a worrisome sign.

14) A) Sideroblastic anemia is the only listed disorder not associated with hyperlipidemia.

15) C) Methanol, when abused, is associated with blindness. Ethanol, administered under medical supervision, is the antidote. However, it is not associated with hyperlipidemia.

16) D) A previous diagnosis of pertussis is difficult to confirm. The duration of protection after infection with B. pertussis is unknown. Therefore all routine vaccinations are indicated despite history of pertussis disease.

17) B) This child has missed his kindergarten dose of DTap, but since he is older than 7 he cannot receive the full diphtheria dose; therefore Tdap is the right answer. Had this child received the booster recommended at Kindergarten entry, then no immunization would be needed at this point.

Answers

18) B) Infants **do** normally cry more during the second month; however, colic rarely occurs after the third month. Crying peaks at age 6 weeks, just when the baby starts to smile and the parents smile as well.

Parental fear and anxiety can play a role in colic, e.g., climbing up the entertainment center.[1,2] Infants can of course cry in response to many things besides hunger. Flexion of the arms and legs are not diagnostic of colic. These symptoms can be part of normal crying or be suggestive of a serious gastrointestinal problem such as obstruction.

19) B) Alcohol consumption is the most frequent problem associated with teen accidents and injuries.

20) B) HIV infection would not be a contraindication for the MMR vaccine and neither would a child with ALL in remission. A child with sickle cell disease or otitis media can also receive the vaccine.

Precautions are suggested with thrombocytopenia and for any child who has received immune globulin within the past 3 to 11 months. Therefore, a child with ITP receiving IV IG should not receive the vaccine.

Other contraindications include pregnancy, history of an anaphylactic reaction to neomycin or gelatin, long-term immunosuppressive therapy, and active hematological or solid tumors.

21) E) This would be a question that falls under the category of "it looks easier than it is". Logically it would appear that unilateral testicle would be a contraindication to contact sports. However, it is not. Wearing a protective cup may be a good idea, nonetheless.

Fever and acute diarrhea with dehydration should be resolved prior to participation in contact sports. Hepatomegaly or splenomegaly could result in a rupture of either organ, and either should be resolved prior to participation.

Any skin lesion, including impetigo that can be spread by direct "contact" would make participation in contact sports contraindicated.

---

1 Such activities are best done away from the home, and away from law enforcement.
2 If the infant-crying to father-whining ratio is greater than 2 you should be concerned.

Copyright 2018 by Medhumor Medical Publications, LLC

22) C) Suicide is the second leading cause of death among adolescents. MVA is the first. While girls attempt suicide more frequently, boys are "more successful," partly because they choose more violent and definitive means. Firearms are the most common method used in "successful" suicide attempts. Only a fraction of all suicide attempts come to medical attention. Television has been shown to increase suicide attempt rates.

23) A) You probably recognize serum gamma glutamyl transferase as one of the liver function tests. An elevated GGT correlates with chronic alcohol abuse, as does an increased mean corpuscle volume. Hypoglycemia, metabolic acidosis, and elevated blood alcohol levels all correlate with acute alcohol toxicity rather than chronic alcohol abuse.

24) E) There is an association between the use of anabolic steroids and the use of other drugs. Teens who use anabolic steroids are more likely to engage in fighting behavior. Teens who abuse drugs in general are more likely to engage in violent behavior, regardless of gender.

25) C) The two most effective tools in preventing tooth decay in the general population are community fluoridation and fluoride toothpaste.

Fluoride varnish application is appropriate for populations at high risk for developing dental caries. The highest identified group is those of lower socioeconomic status due to a myriad of factors. Application of fluoride varnish twice a year is now recommended for this but not the general population.

26) A) Edrophonium testing is relatively contraindicated with infantile botulism and therefor would not be appropriately used in differentiating transient myasthenia gravis from infantile botulism.

The age of onset is important in differentiating the two disorders. Transient myasthenia gravis is usually present at birth and infantile botulism is more acute later in infancy. There would be a maternal history of myasthenia gravis differentiating transient neonatal myasthenia gravis from botulism. Constipation is present with botulism only. Both disorders have excellent long term prognoses when managed appropriately.

Answers

Poisons and Toxins

27) B) The boy in the vignette likely ingested a hydrocarbon. Tachypnea, coupled with wheezing and crackles along with lethargy are typical findings for hydrocarbon ingestion. The initial management would consist of supplemental oxygen as well as a bronchodilator like albuterol.

28) C) When it comes to lead, 5 is the new 10. That is to say, in the past a lead level of 10 micrograms/dL was the lowest level of concern. Today the level of concern has been lowered to 5 micrograms/dL. Calcium, iron and vitamin C actually **lower** the absorption of lead and therefore have some benefit. Unfortunately, the neurocognitive effects of lead toxicity are not reversed with chelation therapy. The neurocognitive effects of lead toxicity unfortunately do included behavioral manifestations such as impulsivity and inattention. As of the publication of this book, annual universal screening of all children is not mandatory. It is however required for all children insured by Medicaid, at age 1 and 2. In addition all high risk children are required to have their lead levels checked. This includes foreign adopted children, refugees, and children whose parents are exposed to lead either at their job or through their hobbies.

29) D) Toxic ingestion of clonidine, lorazepam, imipramine and even iron can lead to **hypo**tension. Toxic ingestion of amphetamines would have the opposite effect by causing **hyper**tension. In fact all benzodiazepines, tricyclic antidepressants and antihypertensive medications can lead to hypotension.

30) C) Patients with amphetamine overdose can present with vomiting, mydriasis/ dilated pupils, fever and hyperreflexia.

In addition they can present with **muscle weakness** rather than increased muscle strength. They can be also be talkative and irritable, if not in a manic rage. Hypertension is common as well. In a severe overdose, coma and/or stroke are possible.

31) D) Hypoglycemia can result from salicylate toxicity due to liver toxicity and impaired glucose metabolism. While **hypo**kalemia may be associated with salicylism due to intracellular shifts of potassium in the face alkalosis, **hyper**kalemia would not result.

Dehydration can occur due to vomiting and insensible loss due to initial tachypnea among other processes associated with aspirin ingestion. Although aspirin in a bygone era was used to reduce fever in children, salicylate toxicity can, ironically, lead to hyperthermia. Watch for clues in the question that a child ingested salicylate so you do not go down the incorrect path of infection when presented with a patient with high fever. One clue could include a child having "wintergreen" breath.

In serious cases, pulmonary edema may result, therefore hypoxia is another potential complication of salicylate ingestion.

Answers

Fetus and Newborn

32) D) Given the SGA status, the best explanation for the jitteriness and the tachypnea is hypoglycemia. There is nothing in the clinical history to suggest asphyxia and bilateral ankle clonus is normal in a newborn. (Despite the perfect clonus rhythm quitting at this point is too risky; you may want to stay in touch and track his career though.) Likewise, sepsis is not likely, especially if IV D10 2-3 mg/kg clears up the problem.

33) D) Ampicillin and gentamicin still remain the optimal combination in the NICU setting to provide coverage for the most common organisms causing neonatal sepsis. They have minimal toxicity and adequate CSF penetration.

The other possibility among the choices would be ampicillin and cefotaxime However this regimen has resulted in outbreaks of sepsis due to drug resistant organisms.

34) B) It is partially water soluble and therefore less reliant on bile acid and micelle formation. It is also broken down more effectively by lipase. Biliary secretion is hampered by chloride channel abnormalities in CF patients. Remember CF patients have difficulty with exocrine function in general.

35) B) You might be tempted to pick C, but that is usually part of the history and only raises suspicions of choanal atresia, but does not confirm it. The pureed sea conch is for recreational purposes only after you have passed the exam.

36) B) This is clearly a congenital infection and given the finding of cerebral calcifications you should easily have narrowed your choices down to A and B. However, "retinal irritation" implies chorioretinitis, which is consistent with congenital CMV. Notice that the question did not specify periventricular or diffuse calcifications; therefore, you need to know other factors that distinguish congenital CMV from toxoplasmosis. Retinal hemorrhages which are associated with child abuse would not be described as "retinal irritation".

37) D) CMV is best diagnosed with a urine culture.

38)
1) (B)
2) (D)
3) (A)
4) (C)
5) (E)

These are the ages when the reflexes listed can be expected to disappear under normal conditions.

The palmar grasp disappears at 4 months.

The plantar grasp disappears at 9 months.

Automatic stepping stops at 2 months.

The moro reflex disappears at 6 months.

The money grasp reflex actually accelerates upon law school graduation, making this a very tricky question.

39) E) Diabetic mothers have a high incidence of polyhydramnios, pre-eclampsia, and pyelonephritis. Infants of diabetic mothers are at increased risk for congenital anomalies, persistent pulmonary hypertension,[3] and polycythemia. **They are not at increased risk for hypercalcemia.**

40) D) The history is suggestive of a ductal-dependent congenital heart disease since the onset of symptoms coincides with the closure of the PDA and supplemental oxygen is of no help. Therefore, the most important next step would be to start IV prostaglandins to maintain a patent ductus. Since there is no evidence of respiratory distress, establishing an airway is not necessary. Indomethacin would worsen the problem by closing the duct.

---

[3] Due to increased smooth muscle in the pulmonary arteries.

Answers

41) E) Persistent bilious vomiting in a newborn is suggestive of obstruction, and therefore abdominal x-ray would be the next step in order to establish a diagnosis and implement emergency surgical intervention.

If an obstruction were documented on the x-ray then additional studies such as ultrasound might be useful in locating the obstruction. Up to two-thirds of infants with bilious vomiting in the first 72 hours of life have idiopathic vomiting that is benign and resolves.

42) A) Serologic test for syphilis (STS) is usually done at the time of delivery, and congenital syphilis does not produce the findings in this infant. Developmental assessment to approximate the extent of this developmental delay, TORCH titers to confirm the etiology of the intrauterine infection, and evaluation of visual acuity are all-important in this patient. In addition, head CT may reveal intracranial calcifications that, if distributed throughout the brain, would be more consistent with toxoplasma infection than CMV infection.

43) E) The greatest risk factor for hepatitis B in children is perinatal exposure to a hepatitis surface antigen-positive mother. Of all the choices listed, a mother who is a drug user would be at greatest risk for contracting hepatitis B.

A mother from a western European country such as Lichtenstein would not be at high risk. Worldwide, the areas of highest prevalence of HBV infection are sub-Saharan Africa, China, and parts of the Middle East, the Amazon basin, and the Pacific Islands. In addition, the Eskimo population in Alaska has the highest prevalence rate.

44) B) The mention of a breech delivery and the fact that the rash is limited to the buttocks is not random. With the breech presentation it is the buttocks that would have been exposed to the birth canal for the longest period of time and therefore it would be an infection contracted during the birth process.

A vesicular lesion contracted during the birth process could very well be due to exposure to herpes; thus, the most likely diagnosis is herpes simplex neonatorum. Even though they note that the mother's history is negative for herpes does not rule out the possibility of genital herpes at the time of delivery. Of all the choices, this is the most ominous and would require immediate hospitalization to prevent systemic spread.

Indurated subcutaneous plaques on the buttocks and lower back would be consistent with subcutaneous fat necrosis, which is a benign self-limited disorder seen in healthy newborns.

Pigmented macules would be consistent with transient neonatal pustular melanosis, a benign eruption often seen at birth.

Flat bluish discoloration over the posterior spine and buttocks would be a mongolian spot and not ominous at all.

45) E) Since the physical findings and the clinical condition are both normal, this would be classified as *"peripheral cyanosis"* or *"acrocyanosis"* and all that would be required would be placement under a radiant warmer; that in and of itself would solve the problem. Had they described *central cyanosis* along with other signs, it would entail an entirely different workup.

46) D) The non-stress test measures fetal heart rate reactivity in response to spontaneous fetal movements. It therefore measures fetal autonomic nervous system integrity. At around 29 weeks and later gestation when the baby moves, the HR should increase at least 15 beats above baseline for 15 seconds or more. This indicates normal activity.

47) C) Abdominal distension past the first 48 hours would be consistent with a lower bowel obstruction requiring a contrast enema to make the diagnosis.

Answers

48) C) Since the genitalia appear normal and there are no other abnormalities described, an endocrinological workup including head CT would not be indicated.

Bilateral breast hypertrophy is a common finding in newborns. It is secondary to elevated estrogen levels late in pregnancy and will resolve spontaneously. The milky discharge is also a common finding and is known as "witch's milk".

An old wives' tale recommends squeezing the breasts to alleviate the problem. This may actually exacerbate the condition and is ill advised, especially in the presence of a freaked-out father. Reassurance is the order of the day in this case.

IV antibiotics would be indicated if mastitis were suspected. Mastitis would present with breast swelling but also erythema, warmth, and tenderness.

49) E) With this question some of the systematic steps suggested for *all* questions would come in handy to reason this out. Since this question contains all of the numbers needed to calculate the anion gap that should be the first step.

In this case the anion gap is 25 (sodium minus chloride minus the bicarb). Since the anion gap is normally in the 12-16 range, in this case we are dealing with an *increased anion gap*.

The question is now reduced to "Which of the following diagnoses are consistent with an elevated anion gap?" and you would correctly identify the one disease with a metabolic acidosis and an elevated anion gap, which is maple syrup urine disease.

Since distal and proximal renal tubular acidoses are distinguished from each other by the *urine pH* and this information is not provided, you can almost eliminate these choices. But what allows you to eliminate these choices with certainty is the fact that the "loss of bicarb is compensated with the retention of chloride," resulting in a normal anion gap with both renal tubular acidoses.

With the PCO_2 of 28, there is clear evidence of an attempt at respiratory compensation for the acidosis. Therefore, there is no respiratory failure. Polycystic kidney disease does not cause metabolic acidosis.

50) **E)** "To suck mec or not to suck mec" is one of the proverbial question that plagues residents and neonatologist through the ages.

Unfortunately the answer and rationale changes with the wind, and if you do not keep up, the mec will hit the fan.

Current recommendations take into account the infant's clinical status rather than the appearance of the mec itself.

Current recommendation do not take into consider the consistency of the meconium. Endotracheal intubation and suction would be indicated if the infant is not vigorous, needs positive pressure ventilation or develops respiratory distress after the initial assessment.

The infant in the vignette is vigorous, therefore no resuscitation is indicated despite the thick meconium.

51) **D)** Given that the patient is asymptomatic, the rash is classic for *erythema toxicum*. The anxiety is misguided since this is a harmless, self-limited rash that appears within the first 1-2 days of life and usually disappears spontaneously within days.

52) **D)** All trisomies, including Trisomy 13, 18, and 21, are associated with a *decreased* alpha-fetoprotein level. Elevated levels are associated with neural tube defects, multiple gestations, and defects in the abdominal wall (bladder exstrophy and omphalocele).

53) **A)** Dietary protein intolerance is a *non* IgE mediated food hypersensitivity to egg, soy and milk proteins. It can present with heme positive stools, vomiting, and diarrhea and in severe cases failure to thrive.

It typically occurs during the first year of life.

Answers

54) B) Hypochloremic, hypokalemic, metabolic alkalosis would be expected in pyloric stenosis. Because of the persistent projective vomiting seen in pyloric stenosis, normal bicarb production is not buffered by hydrogen produced in the stomach. In addition due to volume contraction triggers increased proximal tubular reabsorption of bicarbonate. This leads to metabolic alkalosis.

Chloride is lost through persistent emesis and the lack of hydrogen ions results in enhanced excretion of potassium leading to hypokalemia.

Although congenital adrenal hyperplasia can lead to electrolyte disturbances, hyperkalemia would be the result.

Fluids and Lytes

55)
1) (F)
2) (E)
3) (D)
4) (C)
5) (B)
6) (A)

Explanation: This is another board classic that is asked every year so know it well. Here is the logic tree to make it easy.

If you note low **sodium** but a **normal chloride**, this is **lab error**.

Pseudohyponatremia would have low serum sodium with a high glucose or albumin, mannitol or anything that takes up "serum space" instead of water.

Hyponatremic dehydration includes a low serum sodium in light of dehydration, so an elevated BUN would be expected.

SIADH and diabetes insipidus (DI) are easy to confuse in the line of fire. Remember that **SIADH** results in *fluid retention* and therefore low serum sodium with low BUN and *inappropriately concentrated urine*.

DI is the opposite. This can be thought of as "inappropriate urine production" resulting in high serum sodium and very dilute urine. Keeping these facts straight should make the fluid grid a point grab on the exam.

56) E) **Furosemide** inhibits the reabsorption of sodium and chloride in the proximal part of the loop of Henle. This promotes excretion of sodium, chloride, water, and potassium.[4] Therefore, the answer would be **hypochloremia** and **hypokalemia**, regardless of whether the patient were taking digoxin as well.

57) D) A systematic approach to this type of question makes it an easy one. Clearly the pH is normal, so there is some sort of compensation, eliminating lab error as an option.

With bicarb of 18 you are looking at *metabolic acidosis that has been compensated by a respiratory effort* (tachypnea) to blow off CO_2, thus explaining the PCO_2 of 30.

---

[4] No relation to Don Henley, formerly of the Eagles.

Answers

58) C) This patient is presenting with signs of *clinical shock*. A bolus 20 cc/kg would be the most prudent "next" step. Normal Saline or Ringer's Lactate would be isotonic solutions and most appropriate to treat the hypovolemia this patient is experiencing.

59) A) This concentration for oral rehydration therapy is chosen because it allows for maximal absorption of sodium through or via the sodium-glucose cotransporter. This is an important point that can be frequently tested on the Boards.

60) B) Laxative abuse, diuretic therapy, pyloric stenosis and Bartter syndrome are all associated with metabolic alkalosis

Organophosphate poisoning is associated with *respiratory acidosis*.

61) D) Arteriole constriction, reduced coronary blood flow hypokalemia and hypoventilation are all consequences of severe alkalemia.

However hypocapnia would not be a consequence of severe alkalemia. In fact hypoventilation in response to alkalemia would result in hypercapnia.

62) C) The clinical presentation and lab findings are consistent with a diagnosis of pyloric stenosis and the most appropriate study would be an abdominal, most specifically a pyloric, ultrasound.

63) A) With **heat stress** one would see decreased exercise performance but little else.

With **heat exhaustion** one would see confusion, nausea, vomiting and a core temperature between 100.4 F and 104.

With **heat stroke** one would see a core temperature greater than 104 F.

Genetics

64) **A)** Gardner's syndrome results in supernumerary teeth (i.e., extra teeth). All of the other choices are associated with a delayed eruption of teeth. E is not exactly correct; since most hockey players are missing teeth but not secondary to delayed eruption of teeth.

65) **B)** Intellectual disability. Here is an example where good test taking skills might come in handy. Choices C and E are linked and can be eliminated narrowing it down to 3 choices. See the Treacher Collins (Teacher Calling) section of the Genetics chapter in our main text.

66) **B)** Aicardi syndrome is one of the few disorders that are inherited in an X-linked *dominant* fashion.

Therefore it is an x-linked disease which can appear in females because it is a dominant trait on the X chromosome. Another feature of Aicardi syndrome is an absent corpus callosum.

67) **C)** Trisomy 18 is associated with clenched fist, rocket bottom feet, prominent occiput and horseshoe kidney. It is also associated with overlapping fingers which has a "clenched fist" appearance. Trisomy 18 is not aassociated with punched-out scalp lesions. These are classic in Trisomy 13 (Patau syndrome).

68) **C)** This is an autosomal dominant trait, and therefore all children have a 50% chance of having the disorder, regardless of gender. Don't be tricked by a decoy choice that splits the pattern based on gender. Remember if Mom has the disorder she cannot be a carrier, and the disorder is not X-linked recessive. Noting which parent has the disorder will give you such clues.

69) **C)** Scalp defects, congenital heart defects, microphthalmia, and holoprosencephaly are all seen in Patau syndrome (trisomy 13). Rocker bottom feet are seen with Edwards's syndrome (trisomy 18). Holoprosencephaly, by the way, is a single-lobed brain structure with severe skull and facial defects.

Answers

70) D) 2/3. Here you would have to know that CF is an autosomal recessive disease. Since this is an *autosomal* recessive trait, the gender is irrelevant. Mentioning that this is a sister is therefore irrelevant. Go ahead and toss that red herring aside. The sister is unaffected, so if you run your Punnett square, you will get 3 possibilities for her: 1 possibility is disease free, no carrier and the other 2 possibilities are disease free, carrier, leaving you the answer 2/3 = 66%.

71) A) Wide gap between first and second toe, duodenal atresia, redundant skin on the posterior neck and a transverse palmar crease are consistent with Down syndrome; cleft lip and palate are not.

72) E) Tetrahydrobiopterin (BH_4) is a cofactor for the enzyme *phenylalanine hydroxylase* which breaks down phenylalanine into tyrosine. Therefore tetrahydrobiopterin deficiency can be present with a positive PKU test and clinical deterioration can present even when normal phenylalanine levels are maintained. All documented cases of PKU should be followed up with testing for BH4 deficiency. By the way, A is correct but not the best answer.

73) A) Since this hemophilia A is an X-linked recessive disorder and the father is unaffected, his X chromosomes are also unaffected. Therefore, none of his offspring will be affected and the correct answer is 0%.

125% is the effort put forth by many professional ballplayers when they state "Everyone on this ball club is giving a 125% effort to win".

74) E) This is an example of a disorder inherited through DNA found in the mitochondria (in the cytoplasm as in non-nuclear DNA). This is inherited strictly in a **matrilineal inheritance** pattern. This is easy to remember if they ask any questions on the inheritance of disorders having to do with abnormalities in mitochondrial DNA. **M**atrilineal and **m**itochondrial both begin with **M**.

75) C) This is Prader-Willi syndrome, which may have confused you into choosing E, which is Slick Willy syndrome. Deletion of dad's chromosome 15 leads to Prader-Willi syndrome because of maternal disomy where both number 15 chromosomes come from the mother

When the deletion occurs on the mother's number 15 chromosome the patient has Angelman syndrome because of paternal disomy where both number 15 chromosomes come from the father.

Remember **P**rader is due to **p**aternal deletion and Angel**m**an is due to **m**aternal deletion.

76) C) Tuberous sclerosis is inherited in an autosomal dominant pattern.

77) 1) (B)
2) (A)
3) (C)
4) (A)
5) (C)

Noonan was and is sometimes referred to as "male Turner's". This is a misnomer. Turner's affects genetic females only but Noonan can occur in both males and females. They share *some* phenotypical similarities, but they are quite different. Turner's is X/O (with a variety of mosaic variations) and Noonan syndrome has no identifiable genetic pattern.

78) C) 1 in 150. is the correct answer.

Here you need to know that the carrier rate for CF in the general population is 1/25 (basically the only one you will need to memorize) and that CF is autosomal recessive. The sibling has a 2/3 chance of being a carrier. You can work this through logically using the Punnett Square or you can just memorize it. When 2 carriers get together there is a 1/4 chance of having a child with CF.

Putting it all together you get 1 in 150 as the correct answer to this question.

$(1/25) \times (2/3) \times (1/4) = 1/150$

Answers

Allergy and Immunology

79) E) Children with terminal complement deficiencies (C5-C9) are at risk for all *Neisserial* infections.

80) E) When you see the words **eczema along with recurrent infections and thrombocytopenia**, think Wiskott-Aldrich syndrome.

While *Pneumocystis carinii* pneumonia is commonly seen with AIDS, the eczema and thrombocytopenia makes AIDS less likely.

81) A) Ataxia telangiectasia is an autosomal recessive condition that presents in early childhood with regression of motor milestones. Recurrent sinopulmonary infections involving encapsulated organism is seen.

Immunologic findings include decreased IgA levels as well as decreased IgG levels and T-lymphocyte deficiency. It is associated with an increased risk of malignancy, especially Hodgkins lymphoma and leukemia.

82) E) The most frequent form of chronic granulomatous disease (CGD) is inherited in an x-linked recessive pattern. However the other forms are inherited in an autosomal recessive pattern.

This is a disorder of phagocytic function. It is best diagnosed with the nitroblue tetrazolium test (NBT).

Urinary retention and bowel obstruction are potential complications.

Prophylactic treatment is indicated with trimethoprim/sulfamethoxazole and itraconazole.

Leukocyte Adhesion Deficiency (LAD) is a defect in chemotaxis.

83) E) Oral medications have no role in the immediate management of acute anaphylactic reactions. Appropriate treatment of an acute anaphylactic reaction is epinephrine (1:1000) SQ 0.1 mg/kg.

The steroids are used to prevent a phase II reaction a few hours after the initial reaction.

84) C) The most common trigger for life threatening anaphylaxis in children is food.

Answers

Infectious Disease

85) D) This is consistent with the Jarisch-Herxheimer reaction, in the past more commonly associated with the treatment of syphilis but also seen in the treatment of Lyme disease. It is due to lysis of the organism and the release of endotoxin.

86) A) Of all the drugs listed only ethambutol is associated with optic neuritis.

87) D) The symptoms described are consistent with **cat scratch disease. Bartonella henselae** is the causative agent.

After an incubation period of 7–12 days,[5] one or more 3–5 mm red papules develop at the site of cutaneous inoculation, often reflecting a linear cat scratch. **Chronic regional lymphadenitis is the hallmark**, affecting the first or second set of nodes draining the entry site. Other nonspecific symptoms include malaise, anorexia, fatigue, and headache.

Unilateral conjunctivitis is a common "atypical"[6] finding. Presumably, direct eye inoculation occurs when hands touch the eye after touching a cat.

88) E) Antibiotics are not indicated with "uncomplicated" *Salmonella*. That would apply in this case since the patient is now afebrile and the blood cultures were negative, indicating "non-invasive" disease. Antibiotics would not shorten the duration of the disease and in fact might induce the carrier state.

Antibiotics are recommended only in children at risk for invasive disease. This would include infants younger than 3 months of age. The child in the vignette is 9 months old. If indicated, all of the antibiotics listed except erythromycin would be appropriate.

---

5 Range 3–30 days.
6 Yes, it is described as a "common" atypical finding, and many would argue that this is an oxymoron or a contradiction in terms. But such is life in the "semantic" world of medicine.

89) D) Because of the rarity of subsequent cases and the low risk of invasive group A *Strep* infections, routine prophylaxis is not recommended for school contacts. However, if the child should become symptomatic then a throat culture would certainly be appropriate.

90) A) The mechanism of action of the botulism toxin is to block the release of acetylcholine from the *presynaptic* neuron.

Gentamicin and other aminoglycosides have been known to enhance "neuromuscular blockade." Therefore, gentamicin would be contraindicated in an infant admitted for botulism poisoning. In addition antibiotics in general are not used to treat infantile botulism. Treatment is largely supportive. **Constipation is a very early sign** and often precedes all other signs; *it is not a late finding.*

Last but not least, the active ingredient in Botox® injections is indeed botulism toxin; thus the name "Botox". It is used by plastic surgeons to reduce facial wrinkling. Apparently it does so by paralyzing muscle tissue. So much for function over vanity.

91) D) The only child who would legitimately be excused from school would be the child with *Strep* throat.

In general, a child with *Strep* throat should be kept from attending school until he is afebrile for 24 hours and/or has been treated with appropriate antibiotics for 24 hours.

Asymptomatic Salmonella gastroenteritis does not require exclusion from school.

Infectious mononucleosis does not preclude a child from attending class; the risk for spreading it to classmates is very low.

92) E) Three of the drugs listed are recommended to treat tularemia. However ciprofloxacin has been used effectively in a limited number of cases even though its use has not been approved in children younger than 18.

Doxycycline would not be appropriate in a child younger than 8 due to the risk for dental staining especially in a child when there are alternative medications that are approved in children younger than 8.

Gentamicin would be an appropriate first line medication in this child.

Answers

93) D) Paronychia is the inflammation of the nail bed, or periungual skin.

An *acute* paronychia is often the result of chronic overzealous nail trimming or biting. This would be characterized by redness, swelling, and sometimes purulent discharge.

However, *chronic* paronychia noted in this question would present as edema and inflammation but not necessarily purulent discharge. Chronic paronychia is most likely due to Candida albicans or mouth flora and is often a result of thumb sucking. It is the chronic exposure to moisture that causes the problem.

94) B) Rifampin prophylaxis is recommended for household contacts, especially young children and childcare and nursery contacts during the previous 7 days. Of course, anyone who came into direct contact with body secretions[7] would also be treated with rifampin prophylaxis.

While it won't factor into the exam, you should warn folks on rifampin of the strange electric-orange color their urine will take on. It can stain contact lenses and more importantly can interfere with the efficacy of oral contraceptive pills, anti- seizure meds, and some anticoagulants.

95) A) Don't be so quick to jump on the group A beta-hemolytic *Strep* bandwagon while ignoring the possibility of a "virus", Adenovirus to be exact. Adenovirus is the most likely cause of the above set of symptoms. This is especially so during the summer, and on the exam.

96) D) This is a classic presentation of Staph pneumonia. It initially manifests as upper respiratory tract infection signs and symptoms followed by a rapid progression to signs of more severe respiratory distress and fever. Abdominal signs such as distension can also present. Of important note, the right lung is involved in 65% of the cases and is often accompanied by an effusion. Therefore, the CXR findings alone should serve as a good clue to keep your "Staph" on your right side.

---

[7] Which would include you, the treating physician.

97) B) This is a classic description of staphylococcal scalded skin syndrome. The "clear and shiny areas of denuding" is "Nikolsky sign", where areas of the epidermis will separate with minor force or gentle stroking of the skin. The description of crusted lesions around the mouth and nose is another tip off that *Staph* is the guilty party. Remember that erythema multiforme usually involves mucous membranes and would be described as lesions in but not around the mouth. Easily remembered as erythema multiORALforme.

98) B) The isolation of *Mycobacterium avium* complex would be most suggestive of AIDS in this HIV-positive child. The vignette represents the classic presentation and *is more common in HIV-positive patients who may not have received appropriate antiretroviral therapy.*

By the way, it is diagnosed via isolation in the blood, bone marrow, or other tissue. *Isolation from stool does not necessarily confirm the diagnosis.* Therefore, watch out for trick questions leading you down that path to the wrong pathogen or wrong diagnostic test.

99) C) This is a fairly straightforward clinical description of an osteomyelitis. The most common cause of osteomyelitis is *Staph aureus*. The absence of swelling or effusion on the knee makes septic arthritis unlikely.

100) E) Fecal H. pylori antigen, endoscopy with biopsy, and urease breath test would all be valid tests to establish the eradication of H. pylori following treatment. It is important to note that the stool antigen test may remain positive for up to 90 days after treatment.

H. Pylori IgG would only be helpful to establish if a patient had or has disease making it only useful in research studies.

If the question had asked for the preferred noninvasive test the answer would have been fecal H. pylori antigen.

101) C) All childcare and nursery school contacts during the previous 7 days would require chemoprophylaxis. Since this child was exposed 5 days ago chemoprophylaxis for the child is indicated. However since the parents did not have close contact with the index case they will not need chemoprophylaxis.

Answers

102) **D)** The rash and clinical presentation of a centripedal spread of a papular-vesicular rash preceded by fever is consistent with a diagnosis of varicella or chickenpox.

Direct fluorescent antibody would work off of a sample from the lesion itself and would provide the quickest answer. Viral culture would establish the diagnosis but it would take a long time. Polymerase chain reaction would also establish the diagnosis but is not as widely available as direct fluorescent antibody and therefore would not be the quickest method.

Molecular amplification would be appropriate if the virus cannot be detected by rapid isolation as is the case with varicella. Skin biopsy would be completely inappropriate.

Of course back in the old days varicella/chickenpox was a simple diagnosis made on clinical grounds. However, these are the boards and you are expected to know how to confirm the diagnosis definitively.

103) **C)** The most commonly used antibiotics used for MRSA are trimethoprim-sulfamethoxazole and clindamycin, but these are not listed. Of the antibiotics, listed, doxycycline and levofloxacin would both be appropriate. However, levofloxacin is not approved for routine use in children younger than 18.

Whenever you are asked a question regarding antibiotic choice and are given the patient's age, it is important to note which choices can be eliminated based on the age of the patient.

Methicillin resistant Staph aureus would be resistant to Amoxicillin/clavulanic acid, cefdinir and amoxicillin.

104) **B)** Enzyme immunoassay antigen detection (EIA detection) taken from a nasopharyngeal swab would be the most appropriate rapid test for influenza virus. Polymerase chain reaction and viral cultures would both be appropriate but not rapid.

105) **D)** The least effective antibiotic in treating Listeria is cefotaxime. This is because **Listeria is always resistant to cephalosporins**.

106) C) Changing the diapers or handling the child's laundry is okay with the caveat that washing hands with soap and warm water is done.

However the mother should not sleep in the same bed as the child, no kissing on or near the child's mouth, and no sharing towels or washcloths with the child.

This all stems from the correct assumption that any child younger than 3 is secreting CMV virus in their urine and saliva.

107) D) Both enzyme immunoassay (EIA) and immunofluorescent antibody (IFA) are appropriate tests for confirming the diagnosis of cat scratch disease. Only EIA was among the listed choices and would be the correct answer.

Antigen skin testing is no longer recommended. Polymerase chain reaction is reliable but not widely available.

108) C) The diagnostic test of choice for rabies is reverse transcriptase-polymerase chain reaction.

Prior rabies immunization does not induce CSF antibody to the virus. Therefore the presence of high CSF antibody titers in the CSF supports the diagnosis of clinical disease.

Clearly the presence of high CSF titers cannot confirm previous disease since previous disease would mean death.

Around 20% of cases many have no documented history of exposure.

109) E) The appropriate treatment for a bite from an animal that could be a carrier of rabies would be a combination of passive and active immunization. This would consist of infiltrating the wound with rabies immunoglobulin. This would be followed by providing HDCV the day the wound was inflicted and then on days 3, 7, 14 and 28.

Answers

110) E) While one could argue that A "I am sorry I have to read the question again" is correct, it would not be the best answer. You would have to read the question and more importantly write down what each serum marker means in words.

For example:
    HBsAb = Hepatitis B Surface antibody means the patient is immune
    HBsAg = Hepatitis B Surface antigen is positive with active disease only
    HBcAb = Hepatitis B core antibody is positive with resolution of natural disease

This makes it much easier to interpret. In this case without the surface antigen or core antibody being elevated, there is no evidence of natural disease.

The presence of surface antibody supports immunity due to vaccination, which is the correct answer.

111) C) HSV is *not* transmitted through breast milk. Of course this would not include herpetic lesions located on the breast itself. *Congenital* infection is associated with maternal and fetal antibody against HSV. *Neonatal* infection, on the other hand, is not associated with maternal and fetal antibodies against HSV. In fact, this is one of the ways of differentiating neonatal infections from congenital infections. If neonatal infection is suspected, treatment should be implemented prior to culture confirmation.

Maternal seronegativity *is* associated with greater rates of transmission.

112) D) The presentation is classic for infectious mononucleosis. The fact that the patient was treated with amoxicillin – clavulanate at a" drive by" telemedicine center (which do exist by the way) without confirmation of culture, suggests a diagnosis of infectious mononucleosis / amoxicillin rash.

Scarlet fever is not likely since that rash would be described as sandpaper and generalized, without evidence of spleen enlargement. The gradually enlarged lymph nodes and other findings are more consistent with this diagnosis rather than an acute systemic allergic reaction.

Inborn Errors of Metabolism

113)
1) (D)
2) (A)
3) (C)
4) (B)

PKU is associated with "mousy odor" urine whatever that is. You won't have to actually smell the urine just identify the association.

Urine smelling like sweaty socks is associated with isovaleric acidemia.

Infants with maple syrup urine disease can present with hypertonia and tachypneic during first week of life.

Dark urine is associated with alcaptonuria.

114)
1) (D)
2) (D)
3) (A)
4) (D)
5) (C)
6) (B)

For #2, Both Menkes Kinky hair syndrome and Wilson Disease involve disruption of copper metabolism and both are associated with low serum copper and ceruloplasmin levels. However, total body copper levels are high and are deposited in body tissue in both cases. Only Wilson's disease results in hepatic failure. There is no specific treatment of Menkes kinky hair syndrome (insert your own hair style joke). Treatment for Wilson's disease is D-penicillamine, not penicillin, so remember to read the question carefully.

Answers

115) **E)** Both hereditary fructose intolerance and galactosemia present with vomiting, irritability, and hepatomegaly. Once again, timing is everything. The patient in this question is only 3 weeks old and has been "breast fed". This is the key to the answer and the reason galactosemia is the correct answer.[8]

In addition to seizures, hypoglycemia and cataracts can also be a part of the initial presentation. Elimination of galactose from the diet reverses the clinical manifestations, including the cataracts.

Infants with galactosemia are also vulnerable to gram negative sepsis.

116) **D)** Elevated homocysteine levels are a known risk factor for cardiovascular disease. The mechanism of action is felt to be via damage to the vascular endothelium. Therefore, children with homocystinuria are at increased risk for a cerebral vascular accident. Treatment is aimed at reducing serum homocysteine levels. Sometimes "pyridoxine"[9] supplementation can reduce homocysteine levels; therefore, homocystinuria is the one metabolic disorder that can sometimes be treated with vitamins. This would be a fair question on the exam.

People with Pompe (Pompous) disease have big heads and egos but not necessarily prone to cerebral vascular accidents.

117) **C)** The key to getting the question correct is noting the symptoms began **after** breast-feeding stopped and commercial formula and other food sources were introduced. Hereditary fructose intolerance is due to the deficiency of the enzyme 1, 6-biphosphate aldolase. I wouldn't waste time memorizing this; however, it does pay to know the clinical manifestations. The presentation is of an otherwise healthy newborn that after the introduction of feedings becomes symptomatic. Symptoms can include jaundice, hepatomegaly, vomiting, irritability, lethargy, and even coma. Lab findings include hypoglycemia and the presence of **reducing substances** in the urine during an episode.

The symptoms resemble galactosemia, but the timing is wrong for that. Galactosemia would present earlier on and would occur with breast-feeding or cow's milk formula feeding, but of course, not with soy formula.

---

8 Deficiency of uridylyl transferase.
9 Vitamin B6.

118) C) The physical findings in this patient are consistent with reactive arthritis, previously known as Reiter syndrome, best remembered as someone who can't see, can't climb a tree and can't pee, thus you could expect that he would also be complaining of dysuria as a result of urethritis.

119) E) Of all the conditions listed, soy milk would be most appropriate for a patient with galactosemia. Infants with galactosemia cannot convert galactose to glucose. Therefore, soy formula would be most appropriate. Many infants with cow milk allergy or allergic colitis cannot tolerate soy formula due to cross reactivity.

120) B) The combination of blunted growth and development along with hypotonia, hepatosplenomegaly and a cherry red spot makes for a diagnosis of Niemann Pick disease. Tay Sachs also has a cherry red spot but does not present with hepatosplenomegaly.

Answers

Endocrinology

121) C) Type 2 diabetes (insulin resistant) is being seen with greater frequency in the pediatric age group with an average age of onset of 12-1/2 vs. 7-1/2 for Type 1(insulin dependent). Type 2 diabetes is associated with obesity. Acanthosis nigricans (pigmentation in skin folds) is specifically associated with insulin resistance and is therefore more closely associated with type 2 diabetes. Metformin is an oral agent which decreases insulin resistance and is used to treat Type 2 diabetes. Both type 1 and type 2 are associated with hyperglycemia.

122) E) The most definitive way of distinguishing type 2 from type 1 diabetes mellitus is to measure beta cell autoantibody levels since type 1 diabetes is caused by autodestruction of the beta cells while type 2 is not. While diabetic ketoacidosis (DKA) is more common in type 1 disease it can present in type 2. A family history of type 2 disease would represent a risk factor for the same. However that does not mean a person with a strong family history of type 2 diseases, which is quite common, could not develop type 1 anymore than if they came from a family with a strong history of owning little pink houses.

C-peptide correlates with insulin secretion and could be low at initial presentation in both types and therefore cannot be used to *definitively* distinguish type 1 from type 2 disease.

Acanthosis nigricans is common in type 2, however obese individuals can also have insulin resistance **without having type 2 disease** therefore the presence of acanthosis nigricans cannot even confirm type 2 let alone be the way to definitively distinguish type 1 from type 2.

123) A) According to the American Diabetes Association, a diagnosis of diabetes can be established with:

· 2 hour post glucose challenge of 200 mg/dL or greater
   OR
· A random serum glucose of 200 mg/dL p*lus symptoms*
   OR
· Fasting serum glucose of 126 mg/dL or greater **on 2 separate occasions**
   OR
· Hb A1c of 6.5% or greater

This patient's fasting serum glucose of 110 does not meet the ADA criteria. However his 2 hour post glucose challenge does meet the criteria. A serum glucose of 230 is not life threatening and does not require the immediate implementation of oral hypoglycemic agents. Therefore the initial intervention would be nutrition and lifestyle changes with a one month followup. Waiting for symptoms to appear before treatment would be inappropriate.

124) E) Pubarche is the development of pubic hair, menarche is the onset of menses, thelarche is the beginning of breast development, and welders' arc is seen with professional welders who are hopefully past adolescence although not guaranteed.

While the timing of pubertal development can very from person to person, the sequence should not vary. Full development should not occur in one stage before the onset of the next stage. For example, a patient who experiences full breast development and no pubic hair deserves a workup. Therefore there should be partial thelarche not full thelarche before the onset of pubarche. Remember, menses occurs roughly two years after thelarche and pubarche a few months after thelarche.

125) D) The growth spurt tends to occur later in boys at SMR 4.

126) C) The growth spurt tends to occur earlier in girls at SMR 3.

127) A) Hyperthyroid patients who experience thyroid storm can have liver disease and be jaundiced. However hepatomegaly is not seen. Pretibial myxedema is common in adults but not children who are hyperthyroid. While patients with Graves's disease can be exophthalmic, you may experience exophthalmia when you realize the absence of it does not rule out Graves's disease. TSH will be elevated in patients who are hyperthyroid due to a pituitary cause, but not in those hyperthyroid due to a Graves disease, since Graves disease is due to an IgG antibody, and in this case the TSH will actually be low.

128) C) The onset of puberty in boys in marked by testicular enlargement (as well as elongation and thinning of the scrotum) and this is where the latest model orchidometer comes in handy (no pun intended). Remember for guys it's two buds (testes) getting bigger down low and for girls it's two buds (breasts) getting bigger up top. Please insert you own Budweiser® Superbowl commercial here.

Answers

129) D) Thelarche is the endocrinologists' term for breast budding. This indeed is the first sign of pubertal development in females followed by pubarche (pubic hair) and then menarche 1 – 2 years later.

130)
1) (C)
2) (B)
3) (C)
4) (D)
5) (A)

Delayed bone age and family history apply to both hypothyroidism and constitutional growth delay. Parents of children with constitutional growth delay achieve normal height and the children can expect the same fate. In fact frequently the parent's have a similar history of delayed growth. Normal adult height applies only to constitutional growth delay. Patients with hypothyroidism and constitutional growth delay both tend to have delayed, not precocious, puberty. And finally, neonatal screening checks for thyroid conditions, but constitutional growth delay is a normal variant and therefore not checked for in newborn screens.

131) It is important to take a long hard look at this curve since it can very likely appear on the exam.

1) (B) - **Craniopharyngioma. After surgical correction at puberty, height can be expected to increase.**

2) (C) - Hypothyroid. This curve is similar to craniopharyngiomas' curve; however, if they were to present both on the same graph, the hypothyroid would be the one presenting earlier. Growth resumes at the time of treatment.

3) (A) - Untreated congenital adrenal hyperplasia. These children grow rapidly but if they are not treated, their growth plates will fuse early. Look for a steady incline with a plateau effect early on. Note that the adult height will be shorter than expected based on mid parental height due to early fusion of the growth plates.

4) (D) - Constitutional delay. Here children remain on a short growth curve (unlike with hypothyroid, CAH and craniopharyngioma where they plateau out) but then experience the classic growth spurt.

5) (E) - Genetic short stature. In this case, children are on a short growth curve and stay there. They are "just plain short" and will be short adults.

132) C) This is a description of Turner syndrome, and all of the findings are likely associations except for 45, XXY, which would be Klinefelter's syndrome and not a variation of Turner's syndrome.

133) C) Here is an example where hard-fast rules are not absolute. **One cannot assume that a question involving head trauma or resection involving the brain will always lead to SIADH as the answer.** It is always best to put the lab findings into words in the margins. The best explanation for the *hyperkalemia* would be secondary *adrenal insufficiency*.

134) A) The side effects of daily/long-term steroid use include growth retardation, adrenal suppression, cataracts, osteopenia, aseptic necrosis of the femoral head, glucose intolerance, an increased risk of infection and cosmetic effects. **Memory loss is not a side effect of chronic steroid use.**

135) C) Given the fact that both parents "hover" around 5 feet and assuming that the parents had adequate nutrition in their youth and have reached close to their growth potential, this would be familial short stature or "just plain short". There is nothing in the history to suggest otherwise. If one of the parents had experienced a growth spurt, this would have to be noted in the question. Therefore constitutional growth delay would be a possibility, however in this question this is not noted and familial short stature is the correct answer. A bigger clue is that the child is growing at 5 cm/ year, which is the minimum normal rate of growth for children after age 2 and virtually rules out abnormal growth.

136) C) Of all the choices listed the best estimate of this boy's adult height is the mean parental height **plus** 6.5 cm. For girls it is mean adult height minus 6.5 cm.

Answers

137) **D)** This patient presents with obesity, hirsutism, and irregular menses. This is the classic triad of **polycystic ovary disease (Stein-Leventhal syndrome)**.

Polycystic Ovaries develop when the ovaries are stimulated to produce excessive amounts of male hormones (androgens), particularly testosterone, either through the release of excessive luteinizing hormone (LH) by the anterior pituitary gland or through high levels of insulin in the blood (hyperinsulinemia) in women whose ovaries are sensitive to this stimulus.

Polycystic "obese" ovaries should help you remember to associate obesity with polycystic ovary syndrome.

Obese patients with hypothyroidism and excess steroids (intrinsic or extrinsic) tend to be short, as are ptients with gonadal dysgenesis (Turner syndrome). Patients with Prader-Willi tend to have failure to thrive as infants but obesity after toddlerhood, small hands and feet, and intellectual disability.

138) **A)** Regarding thyroid nodules, the majorities are benign. However, it is more likely to be *malignant* if the patient is a younger than 15. Therefore, it is more likely to be benign in a patient who is older than 15.

When it comes to thyroid nodules, at least, size really doesn't matter. Benign and malignant nodules come in all sizes. Additional factors, associated with malignancy risk include, nodules that are irregularly shaped and/or fixed to surrounding tissue.

139) **D)** **Fine needle abscess formation is considered to be the gold standard for preoperative diagnosis of thyroid in adults as well as children.** Benign findings can avoid unnecessary surgery. The diagnostic yield is very much dependent on the skill of the doctor obtaining the sample and the pathologist evaluating the sample. In addition, size here does matter and it is difficult to obtain a sample from a nodule measuring less than 1 cm.

Follicular adenomas and carcinomas cannot be distinguished by fine needle biopsy and require surgically obtained biopsy sample to determine if the thyroid capsule has been invaded by the lesion.

GI

140) **D)** Small bowel biopsy is the definitive test for gluten sensitive enteropathy. If the question asked for the most appropriate initial step than a *Transglutaminase Antibody* (tTG) measure would be more appropriate.

Another example where reading the question is critical to answering it correctly.

141) **B)** One of the hallmarks of chronic non-specific diarrhea is *normal growth*. In fact, if this is described in the question, circle it; there are few forms of chronic diarrhea in the differential that *don't* affect growth and this is one of them. None of the other descriptions are associated with chronic non-specific diarrhea including flatulence of any kind, let alone to the point of having guests leaving on schedule.

142) **A)** A stool pH less than 5 and positive reducing substances suggest carbohydrate malabsorption, which is not the cause of toddler's diarrhea.

Watery diarrhea and absence of diarrhea overnight with an increase incidence in the morning are all consistent with a diagnosis of chronic non specific diarrhea.

Note that grossly "bloody stools" are inconsistent with the diagnosis. Occult blood may be present due to perianal irritation and/or excoriation from the chronic diarrhea.

143) 1) (C)
2) (F)
3) (D)
4) (E)

Fecal impaction will frequently be presented as left lower quadrant fullness.

Partial small bowel obstruction would present as vomiting, weight loss and anorexia.

Crohn's disease would present as pressure tenderness on the right lower quadrant along with systemic findings such as fever and joint aches.

Mesenteric venous obstruction could be seen in a teenager using oral contraceptives.

Answers

144) 1) (A)
2) (C)
3) (B)

Not only is surgery not curative with Crohn's, but it can also accelerate the reoccurrence process.

Both Crohn's disease and ulcerative colitis are associated with ankylosing spondylitis. Surgery is curative for ulcerative colitis

145) E) Whenever you see signs of **pancreatic insufficiency in an infant coupled with anemia,** think of Shwachman-Diamond syndrome. This is an autosomal *recessive* disorder which presents with poor growth and greasy, foul smelling stools that are characteristic of malabsorption. The pancreatic insufficiency is often transient, and can resolve by age 4.

Cyclical neutropenia is another associated finding. **Skeletal abnormalities** such as metaphyseal dysostosis[10] are also common.

This should not be confused with Diamond-Blackfan syndrome,[11] which also presents with anemia in infancy, but without signs of malabsorption. **The normal sweat chloride tests rules out cystic fibrosis**, another possible cause of malabsorption in infants.

146) E) Radiologic studies would be limited to complicated cases, e.g., blood-tinged emesis or apnea. 24-hour apnea monitoring at home would be obviously useful for infants with apnea, which would not be considered "uncomplicated". Pulmonary consultation would be most useful in infants with pulmonary findings, none of which are apparent in this infant. Observation over time, with relux precautions but no medications, would be indicated in cases of uncomplicated reflux until it resolves, typically by 6 months of age.

147) B) While projectile vomiting, apnea and aspiration pneumonia may all occur with GE reflux, they are not *the most common symptoms*, and poor weight gain is very unlikely with uncomplicated GE reflux.

The most common symptom of gastroesophageal reflux in infants is passive regurgitation.

---

10 Whatever that is but very different than metaphysical dysostosis.
11 Congenital hypoplastic anemia.

148) D) Tocopherol is vitamin E, which is responsible for cell membrane stabilization. Deficiency of vitamin E often results in **red cell hemolysis, particularly in premature infants**. Vitamin E deficiency can also impair nerve cell integrity and can result in neurological symptoms.

149) E) Anorexia, slowed growth, drying and cracking of the skin, hepatosplenomegaly, and increased intracranial pressure can all be the result of excess intake of *retinol*, or vitamin A.

It can also result in carotenemia. Consider diet as the cause of yellow colors in a child that is non-icteric.[12] In these questions they will often describe excess intake of carrots, squash, and other foods rich in beta-carotene. In other words, don't choose until you've seen the "yellow described in the eyes".

150) E) Cyanocobalamin is the formal name for vitamin B12.

Decreased absorbtion may seen with:

- Juvenile pernicious anemia
- Celiac disease
- Methylmalonic aciduria
- Homocystinuria

151)
1) (C)
2) (A)
3) (D)
4) (B)

GE reflux is often a normal finding in newborns; therefore, reassurance is often all that is needed. **Rumination** is associated with emotional deprivation and rarely occurs during the night. **Duodenal atresia** is associated with diminished fetal ingestion of amnionic fluid, resulting in polyhydramnios. It is important to remember that **necrotizing enterocolitis** can occur in full-term infants, and it should be considered when presented with a full-term infant with classic signs of necrotizing enterocolitis.

---

12 This would be evident by yellow-colored skin without yellow sclera.

Answers

152)
1) (A)
2) (D)
3) (E)
4) (C)
5) (B)

Vomiting secondary to a CNS cause can be the result of an *intracranial hemorrhage*, resulting in a rapid drop of the hematocrit.

Gastroesophageal reflux can accompany signs such as posturing. *Sandifer syndrome*, which is not included in the question but could appear on the exam, can present with both vomiting and torticollis.

Rumination is primarily a behavioral disorder; therefore, behavioral interventions can often be the treatment of choice.

It is important to distinguish gastrointestinal cow milk allergy from allergic gastroenteropathy. **Allergic gastroenteropathy** is also termed *eosinophilic gastroenteritis*. Eosinophilic gastroenteritis can present with atopy in addition to weight loss, hypoalbuminemia, and diarrhea.

Cow milk allergy can present with chronic respiratory problems, rhinitis, colic, and even occult blood loss. This can occur in a breast feeding child if the mother is ingesting mild protein products.

153) A) Wilson disease is inherited in an autosomal recessive pattern. It can present with a mixed conjugated and unconjugated hyperbilirubinemia and rarely presents before age 3.

D-penicillamine and trientine are both copper chelators used in the treatment of Wilson's disease. Zinc acetate is also useful by preventing absorption of copper from the GI tract.

154) D) Feeding refusal, poor weight gain, apnea and upper airway symptoms are all complications of GERD in infants.

Anemia could be a symptom of GERD in older children possibly in association with hematemesis but not in infants.

155) D) Delayed gastric emptying is an important factor in the vomiting seen during acute rotavirus infection.

All of the other statements are true. Fomites formation plays a major role in transmission of disease. The rotavirus is quite a sturdy little virus, remaining active awaiting its next victim on porous surfaces especially toilet handles and sinks. That it is why it is worth using a paper towel when opening the door to leave a public bathroom

Rotavirus infection is seen during the colder winter months and *has* been isolated from the respiratory tract. Often respiratory symptoms accompany the GI symptoms. Adults are more likely to be asymptomatic when infected with the virus.

156) A) Abdominal migraines can present as episodic periumbilical or epigastric pain. The pain is acute and can last an hour or more and there is often a positive family history.

It is occurs more frequently in *females*.

157) D) Amylase and lipase levels that are 3 times normal levels are consistent with a diagnosis of acute pancreatitis. Levels two times normal may not be consistent with the diagnosis.

The classic presentation of epigastric pain that radiates to the back is rarely part of the presenting picture. Epigastric pain alone could be the way acute pancreatitis presents in children. The utility of imaging is questionable and a normal abdominal ultrasound does not rule out pancreatitis.

Answers

Pulmonary

158) D) Grunting is a common finding in infants who have pneumonia. Persistent cough is a common finding in children *outside the newborn period*. Coughs due to upper respiratory infection are most prominent at *night* and the younger the child is the more likely the cough is due to pneumonia.

159) E) The most likely diagnosis would be a foreign body aspiration. Keep in mind that on the exam they will rarely describe the precipitating episode. They will usually describe a "sudden onset" of coughing in a mobile toddler and/or localized wheezing, as described in this vignette.

160) E) Asthmatic children should not be discouraged from participating in exercise. *Exercise-induced asthma* can best be prevented with the inhalation of a beta-agonist immediately before exercise. Inhaled albuterol usually affords protection for 4 hours; use of a muffler or cold-weather mask to warm and humidify air before inhalation might help as well, but supplemental oxygen shouldn't be necessary. Inhaled steroids would be a good *preventives long term* measure, but would not be effective immediately prior to exercise. Likewise, montelukast is a good daily maintenance medication for persistent asthmatics, but is not indicated for intermittent asthmatics.

161) D) Tracheomalacia is a frequent cause of respiratory distress in a child following surgical repair of a TE fistula. Tracheomalacia is caused by the collapse of the trachea and larynx and the resultant airway obstruction leads to wheezing with expiration.

The symptoms described are not consistent with the recurrence of a TE fistula, which would present as choking and heavy secretions with feeding.

162) B) Family and personal history of other atopic diseases such as allergic rhinitis and eczema, elevated IgE levels, and eosinophilia, are all risk factors for asthma persisting past adolescence.

However, recurrent viral illnesses would not be considered to be a risk factor.

Many infants develop wheezing with upper respiratory infections in the first year of life. Infants without the above risk factors, tend to "outgrow" their wheezing after their 2nd birthday.

163) C) The key is the "rapid onset". The best explanation for the *rapid* onset of symptoms versus a gradual onset of symptoms would be a pneumothorax.

Pneumothorax occurs in 10%-25% of patients with CF who are older than 10, and the patient in this question would be at risk because he is 15 years old.

164) D) The absence of cough during sleep will almost always be the clue that the cause of the cough is not pulmonary in origin. Therefore, tic disorder and psychogenic cough are possible diagnoses with the absence of cough during sleep.

165) E) This is a classic description of exercise-induced asthma (EIA).

When asthma is suspected, pulmonary function testing (PFT) is the best way to confirm the diagnosis. When EIA is suspected, PFT after exercise is of partcular help. Spirometry pre and post bronchodilator therapy demonstrating revisable airway obstruction is gold standard in diagnosing asthma

166) D) Steroids improve pulmonary function compared with the use of bronchodilators alone with acute asthma. Inhaled anticholinergic agents should not be used routinely since there is no current proof that they provide any benefit.

Routine use of antibiotics is not recommended since most fevers in children with asthma exacerbations are due to viral upper respiratory infections. Studies show that proper use of HFA inhalers with spacers have the same efficacy as nebulized medications.

Answers

167) A) Mild persistent asthma is

- Symptoms more than 2 days a week but not daily
- Night symptoms 1 to 2 times a month

There is only minor limitation in normal activity.

Needs short acting beta agonist more than 2 days a week but not daily.

168) D) Chronic use of inhaled steroids has a minimal, if any, impact on adult height. If "no impact on adult height" were one of the choices it would be correct.

The risk of thrush from chronic inhaled steroid use can be minimized with the use of spacers and mouth rinsing after use.

Chest x-rays in preschool children can be helpful since it is very difficult to perform pulmonary function testing in that age group. Therefore pulmonary function testing is not the most objective measurement of improvement for preschool children.

Children who have symptoms 4 days every week have moderate persistent asthma.

169) D) The incidence of pneumonia is higher in children from lower socioeconomic levels, and in boys more than girls. Fever and cough are hallmark symptoms of pneumonia although clearly not diagnostic. Pneumonia is often diagnosed and treated on clinical grounds and chest x-ray confirmation is not required for treatment. Tachypnea can be a presenting sign but is not required for diagnosis.

Cardiology

170) D) Each of the items listed are causes of non-cardiac chest pain in children except foreign body aspiration, which typically causes unilateral wheezing and acute onset of persistent coughing in a toddler.

Note that on the exam they will not describe any suspicion of FB aspiration other than an acute onset of coughing in a crawling infant or toddler.

171) 1) B
 2) A
 3) C

The **Still's murmur** is due to harmonic vibrations of the left ventricular outflow tract therefore it is **low in pitch and often musical in quality.** Of course one man's music is another man's shrilling noise however you only need to know the description on the exam They won't be playing an MP3 file for you.

The **pulmonary flow murmur** is a **systolic ejection-type murmur** that is higher in pitch than Still's murmur and is **heard best over the upper left sternal border**. It is caused by normal turbulence across the right ventricular outflow tract and pulmonary valve.

The **cervical venous hum** is caused by the normal, turbulent flow patterns at the junction of the innominate vein drainage into the superior vena cava. It is often **present only when sitting or standing.**

172) A) *Paroxysmal hypercyanotic attacks* which are also known as *Tet spells* are a particular problem during the first 2 years of life. The infant becomes hyperpneic and restless, cyanosis increases, gasping respirations ensue, and syncope may follow.

Management would include
1) Placement of the infant on the abdomen in the knee-chest position, making certain that there is no constricting clothing;
(2) Administration of oxygen (although increasing inspired oxygen will not reverse cyanosis due to intracardiac shunting);
(3) Injection of morphine subcutaneously in a dose not in excess of 0.2 mg/kg.
(4) Administration of phenylephrine, IV propranolol, and volume expansion are also appropriate.

Answers

173) E) Despite the normal physical exam which would imply a normal neurological exam this scenario is consistent with a thromboembolus that has dislodged into cerebral circulation. Therefore, a head CT would be the most appropriate next diagnostic step.

174) D) The key here is the word "small". A patient with a **small VSD** has a relatively benign lesion that is amenable to a "normal life". This can be described as a *loud, harsh or blowing; holosystolic murmur heard best over the lower left sternal border and can be accompanied by a thrill.*[13]

While these patients may be at risk for pulmonary hypertension, this can be screened by EKG.

It is also important to note that under the new SBE prophylaxis guidelines patients with VSDs are not given prophylactic antibiotics before surgical procedures.

Overall, patients with VSD do lead a normal life with no limitations when it comes to sports and physical activity.

175) E) Captopril reduces ventricular afterload by decreasing vascular resistance.[14] Another example of a medication that serves as an "afterload" reducing agent is hydralazine.

Digoxin enhances cardiac contractility.

Furosemide, spironolactone, and chlorothiazide are all diuretics.

176) B) A syncopal episode that occurs during exercise must be worked up for a cardiac cause, especially **prolonged QT syndrome**, which can result in sudden death if not diagnosed and managed.

Often there can be a family history of "unexplained" sudden death in a young person.

Treatment is via **beta-adrenergic drugs** and sometimes **cardiac pacemaker** placement.

---

13 Not unlike the one you will experience when you get the question right.
14 If you must know, it does so by inhibiting angiotensin-converting enzyme, thus blocking the production of angiotensin II.

177) **A)** This cardiac cath is consistent with a normal heart. Blood coming across the RA, RV into the PA is desaturated blood on the way to the lungs with a low pressure gradient from the RV to the pulmonary artery.

On the left side the blood returns from the lungs saturated and the pressure gradient across the aorta is akin to systemic blood pressure.

178) **E)** While cholecystitis can present with pain that radiates to the shoulder, the unremarkable abdominal exam in this patient rules this out. There is no evidence for GERD causing the chest pain, and the lack of pain with tactile pressure makes costochondritis unlikely and therefore ibuprofen would not be indicated.

Given the description of the 45 year old father being on a medication to reduce his "triglycerides or something like that", there is a very good chance the father has familial hypercholesterolemia. As such, the chest pain the patient is experiencing may very well be angina requiring a cardiology referral and restriction of all strenuous activity until cleared.

This is one of the rare instances where referring to a specialist would be appropriate.

179) **D)** Of all the choices listed only cyanosis distinguishes a simple atrioseptal defect from total anomalous pulmonary venous return. Remember, the 5 "T"s of cyanotic congenital heart disease are Truncus arteriosus, TGA, Tricuspid atresia, TOF, and TAPVR.

Answers

Heme onc

180) C) Hyperphosphatemia, hyperkalemia, and hyperuricemia are all seen in tumor lysis syndrome. Alkalinization is part of the treatment.

However hypernatremia is not associated with tumor lysis syndrome.

181) B) Reed-Sternberg cells, non tender cervical nodes, elevated white blood cell count, and low lymphocyte count are associated with Hodgkin's lymphoma.

A rapidly growing non-tender abdominal mass is more typical of non-Hodgkin's lymphoma.

182) B) Neutropenia is an absolute neutrophil count less than 1500. Just memorize it, that's the way it is

183) E) G6PD deficiency is an X-linked recessive disorder. The best explanation would be for the mother and father to have both passed on an X gene for G6PD deficiency to their daughter.

184) B) The average period between neutropenic episodes is 3 weeks with each episode lasting several days.

185)
1) (A) Chediak-Hitachi syndrome.
2) (B) Chronic granulomatous disease.
3) (D) Leukocyte adhesion deficiency.
4) (C) Cyclic neutropenia.
5) (E) Shwachman-Diamond syndrome

186)   1) (A)
2) (B)
3) (A)
4) (D)

In **iron deficiency anemia**, the **TIBC** is high. Think of iron binding capacity as trucks to transport iron where it is needed. When there isn't a lot of iron around, as is the case with iron deficiency anemia, there are plenty of truck waiting around and the iron binding capacity is high. Serum iron stores (ie. serum ferritin) is low in iron deficiency anemia.

However, with **anemia of chronic illness**, there isn't a lot of iron around and the trucks also don't have any gas, so they remain in the garage, so the iron binding capacity is low. Since the reserves were there before the illness, **serum ferritin** is high in anemia of chronic illness.

Neither one presents with a low MCV and a low RDW. Iron deficiency is a microcytic anemia and presents with a low MCV, however it has a high RDW. Anemia of chronic illness is typically a normocytic anemia.

187)   1) (C)
2) (D)
3) (D)

Hemophilia A and B are both X-linked recessive disorders. Mucosal bleeds are common in platelet disorders and von Willebrand's disease and not Hemophilia A or B.

188)   1) (A)
2) (B)
3) (D)
4) (D)

Ewing sarcoma is uncommon in African Americans.

Osteogenic sarcoma will often present with a history of trauma to the involved bone, followed by persistent pain. The description of "pain worse at night relieved by ibuprofen" is typical of osteoma osteoid, a benign tumor.

In past years this was described as pain relieved by aspirin. However it seems that finally this has been updated to reflect that the use of aspirin in children has been phased out with 1970s rotary phones.

The last description is of Homer Simpson.

Answers

189)
1) (A)
2) (B)
3) (C)
4) (B)
5) (A)
6) (A)

Diamond Blackfan syndrome (DBS) is a macrocytic anemia is due to an arrest in the maturation of red cells which occurs primarily in the newborn period. DBS is often treated with steroids and does *not* spontaneously resolve.

Transient erythroblastopenia of childhood (TEC) is a normocytic anemia due to the suppression of erythroid production. It is a condition which almost always resolves spontaneously. TEC is seen primarily in toddlers

Both TEC and DBS involve the red cell line primarily.

190) E) With a question like this, which is heavy in the lab data and seemingly irrelevant bits of information, it is important to put the findings into words in the margins. With that information you can systematically narrow down the diagnostic choices.

You should note a **"recent URI"**, normocytic anemia, WBC, platelets, and retic count all within normal limits. No liver or spleen palpated on the physical exam.

With a normal liver, spleen, and retic count, you have *already ruled out a hemolytic anemia-like G6PD deficiency, as well as sickle cell disease.*

The labs are consistent with a **normocytic anemia**. Which *rules out iron deficiency anemia* and thalassemia.

The normal WBC and platelets rule out aplastic anemia.

This narrows you down to two choices: Diamond-Blackfan anemia and transient erythroblastopenia. *Diamond-Blackfan is primarily seen in infants* younger than 6 months. Given the recent URI, presumed to be of viral origin, you are left with transient erythroblastopenia.

191) D) Children with neuroblastoma can sometimes, especially on the boards, present with **opsoclonus-myoclonus**, which are myoclonic jerking and random movements of the eyes described in this question.

These findings combined with the abdominal mass makes neuroblastoma the most likely diagnosis.

192) D) Since this is a *female* patient you should note in the margins that an X-linked recessive disorder is unlikely.

Factor VIII deficiency is an X-linked trait therefore Factor VIII deficiency is already ruled out. The history is, suggestive of *von Willebrand's disease* since this disorder is not sex linked and *can* affect females. Therefore a workup for *von Willebrand's disease* would be appropriate.

The workup would include bleeding time, prothrombin time, partial thromboplastin time (PTT), and von Willebrand's factor levels.

193) E) Any question involving "severe" seborrheic dermatitis coupled with otorrhea would suggest Langerhans' histiocytosis. The additional findings of polydipsia and polyuria suggest diabetes insipidus, another feature of Langerhans' cell histiocytosis.

194) D) Of all the disorders listed, xeroderma pigmentosum has the highest potential for malignant transformation. It is an autosomal recessive disorder, and the underlying defect is in the repair of DNA damaged by ultraviolet light. Exposure to ultraviolet light must be avoided, and vigilance for any skin changes is warranted.

195) C) If one parent had retinoblastoma, then there is a 50% chance that the child will have it. Fifteen percent of the cases are unilateral and hereditary, and 25% of the cases are bilateral and hereditary. Therefore, 40% of the cases are hereditary making it the neoplasm with the strongest familial tendency of the ones listed in the question.

Answers

196) **D)** Abdominal pain, nausea, and vomiting, coupled with the jaundice in a child with sickle cell disease should make you think about gallbladder disease.

Intermittent pain for 5 months, would suggest gallstones as the etiology of the pain.

Therefore, an abdominal ultrasound would be the study of choice.

Gallstone formation with associated abdominal pain is common in children with sickle cell disease.

197) **B)** Although chronic fatigue, extramedullary hematopoiesis and growth retardation could be indications for transfusion in patients with hereditary spherocytosis, the *most common indication* would be *aplastic crisis* induced by Parvovirus B-19.

198) **D)** Hereditary spherocytosis is inherited *primarily* in an autosomal dominant pattern. It is not inherited exclusively in this pattern. In up to 25% of cases it appears as a spontaneous mutation in people with no prior family history.

Make sure you read the question very carefully, if they phrased it as "It is *exclusively* an autosomal dominant pattern" this would not be correct.

By the way, you can remember that it is autosomal dominant by changing SpherOcytosis to SpherDOcytosis, to remember it is autosomal Dominant.[15]

199) **C)** Splenectomy is generally *not* recommended in patients *younger than* 5. Splenectomy carries an increased risk of infection with encapsulated organisms, and therefore is not preferred. Whenever possible, penicillin prophylaxis is preferred, especially in the first 5 years of life when risk of infection is highest. Partial splenectomy has been found to help reduce hemolysis while providing some protection against infection. The risk for infection is *highest during the first few months after splenectomy*.

A splenectomy would be indicated in a patient with splenomegaly if they wanted to participate in sports.

---

15 X- Linked dominant disorders are so rare that it will be difficult to confuse which form of dominant inheritance this represents.

200) D) Cyclophosphamide increases the risk for developing bladder cancer as a secondary malignancy.

It also causes hemorrhagic cystitis the reason why copious IV fluids are given during treatment.

201) D) Erythrocyte folic acid concentration is a better measurement of folic acid level "sufficiency" than folic acid levels.

One must first rule out B12 deficiency since if B12 deficiency is present treatment with folic acid will delay the diagnosis and perhaps lead to neurological sequelae.

202) D) It is easy to be diverted into believing this is thrombocytopenia absent radius syndrome (TA) however in TAR they would have to describe the absence of radius with the presence of a thumb. Since Fanconi anemia can present with hyperpigmented patches, short stature and skeletal abnormalities, this should be an easy diagnosis to make.

203) E) The chronicity of the pain coupled with the description of the multiple cysts should raise suspicions of ovarian cancer making serum markets to rule out ovarian cancer the correct answer.

204) B) The patient in the vignette has a mild upper respiratory tract infection. The lymph nodes are classic "shoddy" lymph nodes seen in children and are a typical normal finding. Certainly it would not warrant a workup beyond reassurance. The grandmother's admonitions are trumped by the normal growth and development.

Renal

205) B) Autosomal-dominant kidney disease is also known as **adult polycystic disease**. The kidneys are enlarged and show cortical and medullary cysts that are primarily dilated tubules. This can be diagnosed with renal ultrasound, IVP, or CT scan. Of all the choices listed, **renal ultrasound** would be the most appropriate initial step in helping to establish a diagnosis.

206) B) Gross or microscopic hematuria in the absence of proteinuria, hypertension, or any other abnormality may just be due to exercise. Therefore, observation and perhaps an activity log to correlate with the episodes of hematuria would be the most appropriate next step in this patient. Hematuria should resolve within 48 hours when the urine analysis is repeated.

207) B) The most likely diagnosis is *benign proteinuria*, or perhaps orthostatic proteinuria, which is the most common cause of asymptomatic proteinuria. An *AM urine protein / creatinine ratio* is more accurate than a urine dipstick. There is no indication of more severe renal disease or a UTI in the lab or clinical findings described.

208) A) Low serum complement levels are seen with post strep glomerulonephritis, membranoproliferative glomerulonephritis, and systemic lupus nephritis. We remember these 3 as "PMS" because you if you had PMS, you would not be in the mood to "compliment" anyone. However, low serum C_3 is not seen with focal segmental glomerulonephritis. Low serum complement levels are also seen in shunt nephritis. You can include this in the PMS mnemonic as well.

In fact, low serum C_3 is only seen in the early stages of disease in acute post strep glomerulonephritis, up to 8 weeks, and always returns to normal. This helps distinguish acute post strep glomerulonephritis from membranoproliferative glomerulonephritis and lupus nephritis.

209) D) SIADH results in fluid retention and **decreased urine output**. Therefore, it will unlikely result in enuresis. On the other hand, diabetes insipidus would be associated with excessive urine output and could result in enuresis. Sickle cell disease can have an effect on the kidney's ability to concentrate urine. Seizure disorders can result in urinary incontinence, and lumbosacral anomalies could impact bladder tone.

You can remember that SIADH is associated with retention of fluid with low urine output by memorizing it as "Syndrome of I am definitely hydrated".

210) C) Hemolytic uremic syndrome does occur primarily during the summer months and more often in pre-schoolers (ages 6 months to 4 years). It actually occurs more frequently in families of **higher, not lower, socioeconomic status,** possibly due to the types of foods consumed. It is seen more often in the Northern US and Canada, so choice E is incorrect.

Please note that *E. coli*, the causative agent, is not exclusively found in undercooked ground meat; it can also be found in cheese, yogurt, and mayonnaise.

211) B) Struvite stones are associated with urinary tract infections with organisms which contain urease. In fact struvite stones form *only* in the setting of infection.

212) A) Inflammatory bowel disease is associated with increased absorption of oxalate. Therefore this patient most likely has an oxalate stone.

213) E) Increased water intake and low sodium diet are the first line treatments for hematuria and stones due to hypercalciuria. Hypercalciuria is aggravated by high dietary sodium intake.

Thiazide diuretics would be considered a 2nd line treatment not first.

Answers

214) C) Hematuria and proteinuria occurring together will always indicate serious renal disease on the boards. This would include a variety of nephritides, Alport syndrome, or post strep glomerulonephritis.

215) E) The most appropriate management would be to repeat the urine analysis since the proteinuria could be transiently associated with the febrile illness.

Other causes of a transient proteinuria which must be factored in include vigorous exercise, dehydration, or stress.

216) A) **Hyper**kalemia is an adverse effect of ACE inhibitors not hypokalemia. The other choices including neutropenia, angioedema, anemia and even dry cough are potential adverse effects of ACE inhibitors in children.

217) D) Chlorhexidine contamination, gross hematuria, alkaline pH and phenazopyridine can all result in a false positive proteinuria on urine dipstick.

A dilute urine, i.e. specific gravity greater than 1.015 can result in a *false negative* urine dipstick for protein.

Watch out for a vignette where you are presented with a urine dip positive for 2+ protein where one of these factors is mentioned. The urine specific gravity and pH might just be included in an avalanche of information, which is why it is important to tease it out and note "dilute urine" or "alkaline pH".

By the way, if you are asked how to confirm or rule out proteinuria, a urine protein to creatinine ratio is the test, not a 24 hours urine collection.

Genitourinary

218) E) The child in the vignette is experiencing primary enuresis that occurs independent of activity or time of day, suggesting an anatomic etiology. There is nothing in the history to suggest diabetes insipidus and nothing on history or physical to suggest a neurogenic bladder. Likewise, there is nothing in the history to suggest giggling incontinence or UTI.

The MOST likely explanation would be an ectopic uretal orifice resulting in dribbling.

219) C) The risk of malignancy in the undescended testis is 4 to 10 times higher than that in the general population. Surgical correction (orchiopexy) does not change the risk of developing cancer of the testis. Boys with a retractile testis are not at increased risk for infertility or malignancy.

Self- examination of the testes is important given the increased risk for malignancy even when cryptorchidism is corrected with orchiopexy.

220) E) The mean penile length during the first 5 months of age in a term baby is 3.9cm and 4.1 cm is well within that range. Therefore delicate reassurance of the father is in order.

221) D) Even though in the real word documentation of bilateral descended testicle may not be correct, on the boards any statement not placed in quotes can be considered to be absolute.

You have a testicle which cannot be palpated in a child with previously documented bilateral descended testicles. The correct next step would be to reposition and re-examine the patient.

Even though rare, reascended testes have been documented, so if the testes cannot be palpated in the scrotum on subsequent visits, referral to urology will be warranted.

Answers

222) D) The question did not mention when her last menstrual period was or if she was sexually active.

Certainly any fertile female presenting with a 2-week history of nausea and vomiting before anything else should have pregnancy ruled out first and foremost.

223) D) True bacterial epididymitis is rare in children. Nausea and vomiting are rarely seen in epididymitis which occurs over days rather than hours.

The blue dot sign is present in torsion of the testicular appendage, NOT in testicular torsion. Torsion of the testicular appendage is treated conservatively with NSAID, warm compresses, and reduced physical activity and does not require surgery.

Inguinal hernia can indeed present with acute scrotal pain and/or swelling.

224) D) The vignette describes a classic varicocele which is more noticeable while standing or bearing down which is how a Valsalva maneuver will be described. It typically subsides while laying down. If you are lucky, they will describe it as a bag of worms (but they probably won't). In the pediatric world, no intervention is needed. In the adult world, treatment would be necessary if it interferes with fertility.

Neurology

225) D) Todd postictal paralysis, hemiparetic seizures, a subdural hemorrhage and hypoglycemia could each explain acute lateralized weakness.

However hypocalcemia would not result in acute lateralized weakness.

226) E) This is most suggestive of infantile botulism. Although it classically occurs with ingestion of honey, on the boards and in the real world there will rarely be a history of honey ingestion. That would make the diagnosis of infantile botulism too obvious. This lack of history is especially true on the boards.

In addition, only 10-25% of cases are related to honey; cases not related to honey are usually in rural areas where there is a lot of soil exposure.

227) E) Treatment of infantile botulism is **primarily** supportive.

Antibiotics are not indicated. Gentamicin would particularly be contraindicated since it is associated with neurotoxicity

While one could argue that this question belongs in the ID section, doing so would tip the answer too easily.

228) A) This is a classic description of **tuberous sclerosis**. Head CT would reveal the "tubers" projecting into the ventricles. The hypopigmented patches are likely to be ash leaf spots and the bump would be a sebaceous adenoma.

Answers

229) 1) (C)
2) (B)
3) (A)
4) (D)

Both infantile botulism and myasthenia gravis can involve the eyes.

Only myasthenia gravis would present with a progressive onset. Infantile botulism would present with a more acute clinical picture.

Myasthenia gravis is managed but not cured.

Infantile botulism only requires supportive care but this would be curative. The patient should have no residual effects.

Neither myasthenia gravis nor infantile botulism is prevented with immunization.

230) 1) (B)
2) (C)
3) (A)

A headache that is exaggerated by sneezing, coughing, or straining would suggest the increased intracranial pressure associated with a space-occupying lesion or **structural headache**.

Cyclic vomiting and recurrent abdominal pain also are frequently considered **migraine variants**.

Tension headaches are due to muscle tension or muscle contraction. Tension headaches are often described as feeling like a band around the head or occasionally as pain in the neck or shoulders

231) A) With the focal findings of "mild lower extremity hyperreflexia" coupled with the early morning vomiting and headaches, the past history of migraine headaches would not be a factor in managing this patient at this time.

An MRI of the head to rule out a space-occupying lesion like a tumor is the most appropriate next step.

232) A) The average head circumference of a full-term infant at birth measures 34–35 cm.

Therefore a head circumference of 40 cm in a full term newborn would represent macrocephaly. No other conclusions can be drawn given the information provided in the question.

233) C) When presented with a neonatal seizure, don't reflexively go down the well-trodden path of ischemic encephalopathy. The EEG pattern described is typical of **pyridoxine dependency**, a rare autosomal recessive disorder.

234) E) The combination of an infant with descending paralysis,[16] ptosis, and constipation makes for the classic presentation of infantile botulism.

Myasthenia gravis also commonly involves ptosis, but these patients have worse symptoms in the morning and improve as the day goes on, and **Werdnig-Hoffman** disease typically presents with hypotonia and tongue fasciculations.

Muscular dystrophy presents in toddlers, not infants. Poliomyelitis is often asymptomatic, or may have nonspecific symptoms of low grade fever with sore throat. 1% of patients progress to a asymmetric acute flaccid paralysis with areflexia.

235) D) The combination of diplopia, tinnitus and vertigo in a context of intermittent occipital headaches is a classic description of basilar-type migraine headaches. Patients are fine in between episodes and the neurological exam in unremarkable.

236) C) Regular sleep, exercise, biofeedback and stress management all are recognized as methods to reduce the frequency and severity of migraine headaches.

However an elimination diet which refers to the wholesale elimination of a list of foods is not recommended. It is more prudent to make a list of foods which can potentially trigger a migraine headache and note if there is a temporal relationship.

---

16 Remember to write what is being described in the margins.

Answers

237) C) This is a classic description of medication overuse headaches which were previously known as rebound headaches. This is a result of the overuse of analgesics which shut down the bodies own endogenous response to headaches. Analgesics should not be used more than a couple of times per week.

If more pain management is required then *prophylactic migraine medications* would be indicated including:

> Periactin
> Tricyclic antidepressants such as amitriptyline
> Calcium channel blockers
> Beta blockers
> Anticonvulsants

238) D) The clinical vignette is classic for **absence seizures**. The EEG pattern for absence seizures would be a 3 per second generalize spike and wave pattern.

Appropriate treatments would be ethosuximide, lamotrigine or valproate.

Carbamazepine makes absence seizures worse.

This can be remembered by picturing somebody with a petit mal seizure in the middle an amusement park bumper car park getting "bammed by a car" (carbamazepine)

The clinical description is not consistent with ADHD and therefore neither atomoxetine nor methylphenidate would be appropriate treatment options.

239) B) The ketogenic diet (high fat, low carbohydrate) has been shown to be effective in managing infantile spasms. In addition, adrenocorticotropic (ACTH) hormone, valproic acid and topiramate are all considered first line treatments of infantile spasms.

240) A) Valproic acid, lamotrigine, topiramate and levetiracetam would all be appropriate choices for treating a generalized, non-focal, non-absence seizure in children. Phenytoin has fallen into disfavor in children due to the potential for gingival hyperplasia.

241) C) Carbamazepine would be the most appropriate anticonvulsant for treating complex partial seizures in children. You will likely be presented with a classic vignette with features that include, sudden onset of loss of awareness with a glassy stare, automatisms including lip smacking followed by a postictal period lasting 1 hour or longer.

242) A) Ethosuximide would be the most appropriate treatment for children with absence seizures.

Absence seizures could be described as a lapse of attention with eyes fluttering. They might describe lip smacking but they *resume attention immediately with no postictal period.* They may stop moving but *will not fall*.

Answers

Musculoskeletal

243) C) That is because the combination of recent URI, the ability to elicit some passive movement, low WBC and ESR with only "fluid" being found on ultrasound all suggest toxic synovitis which is self limited requiring no other intervention or treatment.

244) D) Since this is "internal tibial torsion", it should resolve by school age without any intervention in the vast majority of cases.

245) E) **Osteoporosis** is what is being described in the clinical vignette, i.e., fragility of the skeletal system and a susceptibility to long bone fractures from mild or inconsequential trauma. *Osteogenesis imperfecta (OI) is the most common genetic cause of osteoporosis.*

In **achondrogenesis** you would see a severe lack of skeletal development, which is typically detected in utero or after a miscarriage.

Very short limbs, a short neck, and a long, narrow thorax characterize **thanatophoric dysplasia**; also, a large head with midfacial hypoplasia is dominant. They do not have the tendency to fracture.

Juvenile osteochondroses are a group of disorders in which the main features are noninflammatory arthropathies. It would not account for the clinical picture described.

Trifecta imperfecta would be various broken bones secondary to having recommended the horse that came in last to the wrong people.

246) E) These findings are consistent with "nursemaid's elbow", a common injury in toddlers. There is often a history of a caretaker pulling on the arm, perhaps as the child steps off a curb or in various other situations. Watch out while swinging your child around in windmill fashion.

There is no evidence of an infection in the vignette, and radiologic studies are rarely helpful in making the diagnosis. Supinating the forearm while the elbow is flexed is curative and diagnostic; it is one of the most dramatic results in pediatrics.

This condition may reoccur as a result of an injured, stretched joint capsule, particularly if the parents wait to obtain medical treatment.

247) D) Pain described just below the knee over the tibial tubercle in an active adolescent in the absence of trauma and other physical findings is consistent with a diagnosis of Osgood-Schlatter.

Osgood-Schlatter is due to microfracture of the proximal tibial epiphysis where the patellar tendon inserts.

In the past rest was the treatment of choice. Since the risk of avulsion is so small, removal from sports is no longer recommended. The new recommendation is to play through. Physical activity is limited only if the pain gets severe. Ice and pain management is usually prescribed

With *patellar dislocation* there would be more pain noted, especially with palpation of the patella.

Osteochondritis dissecans occurs when the bone adjacent to the cartilage becomes avascular and separates from the underlying bone. The *knee pain is vague*. If the boy had *osteochondritis dissecans* he would probably have an effusion with palpation of the affected area when his knee is in a flexed position. In addition, the pain is "activity–related," with swelling and "catching and locking" of the knee.

248) D) The loss of physical function in the absence of organic illness suggests a diagnosis of **"conversion disorder or reaction"**. Additional history is needed to make this psychiatric diagnosis of exclusion. It is via a good history that the "precipitating" environmental event will often be uncovered.

The elicitation of deep tendon reflexes in a paralyzed leg in this case is the key to the correct answer. Another example of a conversion reaction might be *hysterical blindness* with normal pupillary response to light. Being cognizant of these classic presentations will help you "convert" an incorrect answer to a correct one.

Answers

249) B) After one year of age, the development of blood vessels that extend from the metaphysis to the epiphysis disappear. After that point, the risk of both osteomyelitis and septic arthritis developing the same area is reduced.

250) C) Clubfoot would present with the inability to dorsiflex the foot which is not seen with metatarsus adductus.

251) A) Scoliosis is defined as a spinal curvature greater than 10 degrees on a **posterior-anterior** x-ray.

252) A) The absence of dystrophin results in muscle sarcolemma instability. This leads to membrane instability which leads to muscle damage and poor muscle function.

253) B) Mothers of an isolated case of Duchenne muscular dystrophy where there is no prior family history and the molecular genetic studies in the patient are negative is closest to 10%

Why you might ask? The answer is, this is due to a germline mosaicism. However that is not what you might be tested on. The 10% recurrence risk is something you might be tested on.

254) A) Congenital talipes equinovarus or club foot is best diagnosed cribside by physical examination.

255) D) This should be an easy question. You would not want to correct club foot when the child begins to walk. Let's face it that might impede the child's ability to learn to walk.

Just prior to entering school would be a bad time to correct a foot deformity that prevented a child from walking. During pubertal development teens have enough problems looking like a microphone stand with a head, without having had a lifetime of walking on club feet. Once the growth plate fuses, adult height has been reached. Damage to self image might be quite impressive at that point.

256) C) The most appropriate and least invasive test to order when trying to rule out a muscular original of a child who is hypotonic. Once it is determined that the serum creatinine kinase levels are elevated, you then order further testing to narrow down the specific disorder.

… Answers

Dermatology

257) B) While erythema marginatum is a rare manifestation of rheumatic fever, of all the rashes listed it is most associated with rheumatic fever. It is also one of the 5 major Jones criteria. It is a transient red macule that spreads and is characterized by central clearing.

258)
1) (D) - Erythema multiforme
2) (C) - Erythema infectiosum
3) (E) - Erythema migrans
4) (B) - Erythema nodosum
5) (F) - Erythema confusiosum. (It is difficult to keep these straight, isn't it.)
6) (A) - Erythema marginatum.

Erythema multiforme's involving the mucous membranes is an important component to making the correct diagnosis.

Erythema infectiosum is the formal name of Fifths disease which is caused by parvovirus B 19.

Erythema chronicum migrans is the rash seen in 70% of cases of Lyme disease.

Erythema nodosum is associated with inflammatory bowel disease.

Erythema confusiosum is what you are experiencing right now, which is eyes glazed over trying to determine which erythema is correct on the Exam-ema.

Erythema marginatum is erythematous macules on the back associated with rheumatoid arthritis.

259) C) While erythema nodosum is not unique to tuberculosis, of all the rashes listed erythema nodosum is the only one associated with tuberculosis. Erythema nodosum is characterized by tense, painful nodules found on the skin over the tibia. These nodules are usually purple in color. They can also be seen in inflammatory bowel disease and several other infections, including strep and fungal disease.

260) E) While periungual fibromas and café au lait spots can be seen in tuberous sclerosis, they are not seen as consistently as ash leaf macules. Ash leaf macules are seen in 90% of the cases. Again, reading the question carefully would be critical here.

For those of you who do not frequent mountain terrain and are unfamiliar with what the leaf of an ash tree looks like, the image to the right is what we came up with. Your best bet is to look this up in an atlas. It is basically a well-demarcated area of hypopigmentation.

Other cutaneous lesions associated with tuberous sclerosis include **facial angiofibromas**, which are fleshy growths seen around the nose or cheeks. It is a classic image tested in the picture section of the certification exam. Another lesion is the **shagreen patch**. It is typically described as a roughened raised lesion with an orange peel consistency,[17] seen above the belt line or the lumbosacral area.

261) A) The rash described is seborrheic dermatitis. It typically appears during the first two months of life. It can also appear on the scalp, cheeks, and forehead. It requires no intervention and will resolve over several weeks. Therefore, parental reassurance is the correct answer.

Of course in the clinical world pediatricians frequently might treat mild cases with Nizoral shampoo, and possibly a mild topical steroid. However for purposes of the exam mild seborrheic dermatitis in a 6 week old would not require intervention.

262) B) This rash is due to zinc deficiency. The tip-off should be that the infant is a former premie. Premature babies are at risk for zinc deficiency due to high requirements, decreased zinc stores, and inadequate zinc in hyperalimentation nutrition.

In addition to the typical rash, zinc deficiency also results in irritability and diarrhea. Another disorder worth noting is *"acrodermatitis enteropathica"*, which is an autosomal recessive disorder that results in the impaired GI absorption of zinc.

---

17   The origin of this word is for "shagreen leather" which has an orange peel texture. It would make more sense to call it an orange peel patch, since there are probably only two doctors out there who have actually heard of shagreen leather.

Answers

263) 1) (C)
2) (B)
3) (E)
4) (A)
5) (D)

Tinea capitis, which is a highly contagious fungal infection of the scalp (ringworm of the scalp), can manifest with inflammation and black dots. The black dots are actual stubs of broken hairs.

Alopecia totalis is, of course, Latin for "total hair loss", and this would include the loss of eyebrow hair.

Trichotillomania is caused by compulsive pulling and/or twisting of the hair until it breaks off, resulting in incomplete patches of hair loss and the resulting *moth-eaten appearance.*

Alopecia areata is characterized by the complete loss of hair within well-defined round patches and is of a non-infectious etiology. Although unconfirmed, it is felt to be an autoimmune disorder.

Alopecia neurotica is the total, partial, or incomplete hair loss resulting from the stress of preparing for the board exam; *sometimes* the hair returns. When the hair *does* return, the volume that returns is directly proportional to the exam score; there is no other cure.

264) C) This is most likely post-*Strep* glomerulonephritis secondary to a cutaneous infection due to a nephritogenic strain of *Strep*. The U/A will help establish the diagnosis by the presence of RBCs and RBC casts. Unlike rheumatic fever, the evidence that antibiotics prevent glomerulonephritis is unclear.

265) A) The description of the "one spot" as the starting point is the tip-off that pityriasis rosea is the diagnosis. This spot is called the "herald patch". While a herald patch can often be confused with tinea corporis, it would test negative on KOH preparation. They may also describe the rash distribution as a "Christmas tree" pattern.

266) D) All of the choices with the exception of toxic epidermal necrolysis (TEN) are associated with a bacterial exotoxin. TEN is a "hypersensitivity" reaction and involves full-thickness necrosis of the epidermal layer and deeper. This often results in pronounced erythema, which would also help distinguish this on the exam.

267) C) Given the description and distribution of the rash and the fact that the mother has a similar rash, the diagnosis is scabies. While antihistamines would be part of the treatment, it would not be the "most definitive" therapy for this condition. Always read the question, especially the last sentence, which contains the phrase indicating exactly what they are asking.

Answers

Rheumatology

268) A) It is important to remember that it is **arthritis** which is one of the Major Jones criteria and **arthralgia** one of the minor criteria

Likewise, erythema chronicum migrans is associated with Lyme disease; erythema marginatum is associated with rheumatic fever.

If you had known either of these facts this question is a slam dunk.

269) D) Kawasaki disease is more common in Asian populations and among females. It is more commonly seen in the winter and spring than in the summer and fall.

IV gamma globulin is given during the acute phase to reduce the risk for coronary artery disease.

Most cases of Kawasaki are seen in children younger than 4.

270) D) Thrombocytopenia is not associated with HSP and anaphylactoid purpura is just another name for HSP.

271) C) This is the classic history and physical findings for **bacterial endocarditis** and also an example of when "reading the question" is critical. You might be tempted to choose D but remember that blood culture, not cardiac echo, confirms the diagnosis of bacterial endocarditis. Remember in clinical practice they may ask you to choose between two studies you would conduct simultaneously; however, on the exam you will need to choose the "definitive test" or the one you would do first.

272) E) Each of the symptoms described are consistent with an initial case of rheumatic fever except answer choice E, which is consistent with a diagnosis of Kawasaki disease.

273) B) High fever, thrombocytosis, sterile pyuria, hydrops of the gallbladder and conjunctivitis can be seen in patients with Kawasaki disease. *Bacterial* meningitis is not associated with Kawasaki. *Aseptic* meningitis, on the other hand, can be seen in Kawasaki disease.

274) D) Of the all the symptoms listed only palmar erythema is associated with **systemic lupus erythematosus.**

275) C) Renal involvement occurs in 75% of patients with lupus usually within 2 years of diagnosis and is a major cause of morbidity and mortality.

276) D) Maternal Anti-Ro is the antibody most associated with the development of congenital heart block in newborns.

277) D) The most susceptible racial group for developing lupus are Native Americans; African-Americans are second.

20% of all patients who have lupus are diagnosed before adulthood, usually during adolescence. Diagnosis is rare in patients younger than 5.

After puberty, the female male ratio *increases* from 3:1 to 9:1.

Answers

278) A) The most common sign of early **localized** Lyme disease would be a single erythema migrans (EM) rash at the site of the tick bite. Read the question carefully, the most common sign of **early disseminated** Lyme disease would be EM rash on multiple sites. Myalgia, headache and fatigue would be part of the presentation of early disseminated Lyme disease but it is not part of the presentation of localized disease.

Please note myalgia, headache and fatigue are not even the most *common* presenting signs for the early disseminated disease. That distinction falls to EM rash at multiple sites. Therefore this would be the correct answer if they had asked for the most common presenting sign for early disseminated Lyme disease.

279) A) Bilateral non-exudative conjunctivitis, diffusely erythematous oropharynx, red fissured lips and strawberry tongue are all common manifestations of Kawasaki disease

Discreet oral ulcers and tonsillar exudate are not seen with Kawasaki disease. More than 90% of patients with KD have bilateral non-exudative conjunctivitis so watch for this when they describe any child with several days of high fever.

Ophthalmology

280) **D)** Children with congenital ptosis present with eyelid droop that is often unilateral and results in their lifting their head to see. It is due to an abnormality of the levator muscle and can be corrected surgically. The child in the vignette does not have signs of amblyopia, although this can develop if the ptosis causes vision loss and is not corrected surgically.

There is no evidence of vernal, nocturnal, neurotic or any type of conjunctivitis here. The lifting of the head might be perceived as behavioral if, while lifting his head the child challenged the teacher by saying "You talking to me?" ... "You got something to say? ". Alas this was not described in the vignette, ruling out choice A.

Horner syndrome involves other signs beyond what was described and they would not have pupils that are equal and reactive and therefore choice E is ruled out.

281) **E)** The combination of right sided eyelid droop and right pupil that is sluggish to react to light, suggests a diagnosis of Horner syndrome. The matted hair on the left side, confirmed by the parents to be chronic, suggests right sided anhydrosis, or lack of sweating on the right side which is also consistent with Horner syndrome.

Kings lead hat syndrome is something we made up. It is actually the name of a song by Brian Eno, which is also an anagram for the 80's band "Talking Heads"

Congenital ptosis would only present with ptosis and possible amblyopia if the ptosis is severe and not corrected early enough. There is no evidence of myasthenia gravis which would present with fluctuating weakness of the eyelids and extraocular movement limitations leading to diplopia.

282) **B)** Congenital cataracts can be associated with maternal hypoparathyroidism. They are not associated with maternal hypothyroidism, hyperthyroidism, or hyperparathyroidism. Congenital cataracts are associated with galactase deficiency leading to galactosemia. They are not associated with lactase deficiency.

Answers

283) D) The clinical vignette is a clear cut description of a corneal abrasion most likely sustained by a grain of sand that resulted in the patient scratching and rubbing the eye. Since there is no foreign body noted, the grain of sand likely washed out. The preferred treatment of choice is an antibiotic ointment such as erythromycin without patching. Ointment is preferred to drops since they are more soothing and lubricating. A patch does not aid in resolution and is poorly tolerated by children. If a foreign body remains, the pressure of a patch might even worsen the abrasion.

284) C) The infant in the vignette most likely is experiencing nasolacrimal stenosis or a blocked tear duct. This is suggested by the trickling down of the tears to the left cheek and the accumulation of mucoid material. The latter doesn't necessarily suggest and infection and therefore neither oral nor topical antibiotic ointment is indicated. Since erythromycin ointment was applied at delivery and the neonatal history was described as being unremarkable, gonococcal conjunctivitis is highly unlikely. Therefore the correct answer is instructing the mother on massage technique to unblock tear duct.

ENT

285) D) The presentation is consistent with laryngomalacia, which improves with time and no intervention. Improvement occurs as the cartilage becomes stronger. Think of laryngomalacia when they describe stridor which improves on expiration.

286) C) Tympanic membranes may appear erythematous any time a child is febrile or screaming. Therefore, pneumatic otoscopy is necessary to diagnose otitis media.

287) D) *Epiglottitis* would be an example of "supraglottic" obstruction, which can present with drooling due to the diminished ability to swallow saliva. This is typically due to H. flu and is quite rare due to the success of the HiB vaccine. However like all other diseases eradicated through immunization, it can creep its way onto the boards where most patients are not immunized.

Epiglottitis can be a surgical emergency since the airway can rapidly close off. In general, the obstruction above the glottis improves **with expiration**, but can close down with inspiration since the negative pressure pulling down can collapse the airway. *Therefore, stridor on inspiration* which improves with expiration should make you think of a supraglottic airway obstruction.

A retropharyngeal abscess classically presents with a "hot potato voice" and is another example of supraglottic airway obstruction.

288) A) **Bacterial tracheitis is an acute bacterial infection of the upper airway and does not involve the epiglottis.** However, like epiglottitis and croup, bacterial tracheitis is capable of causing life-threatening airway obstruction. Typically, the child has a brassy cough, apparently as part of a viral laryngotracheobronchitis. *Bacterial tracheitis is often a secondary infection.* High fever and "toxicity" with respiratory distress may occur immediately or after a few days of apparent improvement.

Answers

289) E) Usual treatment for croup (e.g., mist, intravenous fluid, aerosolized racemic epinephrine) is ineffective. Intubation or tracheostomy is usually necessary. Initially, removal of secretions may provide some relief, but ultimately intubation is necessary. **IV antibiotics** are also necessary.

290) D) It is important to realize that they will rarely refer to *laryngotracheitis* as "viral croup". They will either describe it clinically or go by the infinitely more confusing name *laryngotracheobronchitis*.

In addition to the typical "barking cough", some of the more important features to note are the typical age of onset of 12 months, the fact that the stridor is biphasic[18] and that the condition is often preceded by a URI, and the fact that there can even be a "lower respiratory wheezing" component to the respiratory distress. The latter is important to note so you are not fooled if they throw this into an otherwise typical description of viral croup.

An important similar diagnosis in the differential would be ***spasmodic croup***. This is more of an allergic phenomenon, and there is **no seasonal variation**. As with spasmodic croup, there will be no fever and more of an abrupt onset with no preceding URI.

291) A) All of the above can be responsible for *acute otitis media with effusion* with the exception of *Haemophilus influenza type B*. This is sort of a trick question[19] since, thanks to the Hib vaccine, it is the "nontypeable" species that of *Haemophilus* influenza that can cause acute otitis media with effusion. Again, it pays to read the question very carefully.

292) B) These lesions are indeed acquired during the birth process when the mother has vaginal condylomata. Surgery is not curative at all, and repeated laser excision is often needed when the lesions grow back after excision. They are not considered true neoplasms, but may become malignant over time. Malignant degeneration is actually more likely *after* radiation treatment.

---

18 Both an inspiratory and expiratory component.
19 Not unlike that you might encounter on the exam.

293) A) Inflammatory mediators play an important role in persistent middle ear effusion following otitis media infections. As a result, *increased* (rather than decreased) blood flow to the mucous membranes plays a role. Persistent infection is not usually a factor, and myringotomy tubes may be indicated if the effusion leads to recurrent ear infections or hearing loss.

294) D) The key words here are **firm, non-tender** and **several months' duration** (rather than acute onset). This virtually rules out the infectious etiologies listed, including paramyxovirus, which is the name mumps goes by when it wants to impress more exotic viruses at viral cocktail parties. Neoplastic disease is the correct choice.

There is no such thing as psychogenic adenopathy.

295) C) Although it is rarely seen in clinical practice anymore, you must still be familiar with the clinical scenario of *Haemophilus* influenza epiglottitis. Let's face it; mumps and measles are also quite rare these days, yet they frequently appear on the boards. This is especially true in this case where they note that the child has not been immunized.

The combination of stridor, high fever, apprehension, and drooling makes epiglottitis very likely and therefore warrants the presence of an anesthesiologist familiar with intubating children under difficult situations (i.e., a swollen epiglottis). Patients with epiglottitis should be intubated in the OR by an anesthesiologist with ENT or pediatric surgery on standby.

296) A) Daily antibiotic prophylaxis has fallen into disfavor with growing concerns over development of pneumococcal resistance.

297) D) Clindamycin would be the best alternative antibiotic in a penicillin allergic 4 year old with a dental infection.

Answers

298) D) Vomiting and blurred vision would be a sign of suppurative intracranial complication and spread. This should be pretty straightforward and certainly fair game on the exam.

299) E) Evacuation of the hematoma would be top priority to prevent subsequent deformity of the pinna.

300) C) Of all the bacteria listed, Staph aureus is the most likely cause of chronic sinusitis. S pneumoniae and Moraxella catarrhalis can cause chronic sinusitis but they are not the most likely cause.

Nontypeable *H. influenza* can also cause chronic sinusitis, but not *H. influenza* type b.

301) C) Another episode of otitis media in the past 3 months would make withholding of antibiotics inappropriate according to the SNAP protocol.

Additional criteria that make withholding of antibiotics inappropriate would include fever or symptoms of otitis media for more than 48 hours. Chronic conditions which might impede an immune response, toxic appearance, evidence of perforation or impending perforation.

Additional contraindications include poor parental understanding of the protocol and/or difficulty gaining access to a medical facility afterward.

302) D) The right sided heart sounds coupled with recurrent sinopulmonary infection suggests a diagnosis of Kartagener's syndrome or cilia dysmotility syndrome and electron microscopic exam of the nasal mucosa would be most helpful in establishing the diagnosis.

303) B) Of all the choices only choice B, saline washes have been shown to be effective, for managing nasal congestion and mild sore throat in children with upper respiratory tract infection caused by rhinovirus.

Oseltamivir is only effective against influenza virus if caught in the first 48 hours of infection. **Guaifenesin** has not been shown to be effective to increase or decrease cough frequency and clearance in children. Inhalations of steam, the basis of chicken soup therapy has not shown to reduce rhinovirus replication or viral titers in nasal secretions. However, no harm in serving up a hot bowl of chicken soup when you are not feeling well!

304) E) It is important to realize that when you are presented with a recently removed tick or a situation where the doctor removed the tick the risk for Lyme disease is very low and therefore reassurance will be the correct answer. Paradoxically it is the tick bites that are not noticed, which are at highest risk for developing Lyme disease.

Therefore no tick is high risk on the boards. Watch for a presentation where there is **no** history of a tick bite with a clinical history consistent with Lyme disease. Workup and/or treatment for Lyme disease would be very appropriate in these cases.

305) B) The patient in the vignette presents with clear rhinorrhea that is pruritic to the point that she rubs her nose red. In addition, she is sneezing a lot. The dead giveaway is the swollen blue turbinates.

If you did not realize the bluish-tinged turbinates are associated with allergic rhinitis then you "blue" this question. Additional "blue" findings could have been bluish lower eyelid swelling, which are the classic allergic shiners. In addition, to the red nose we could have described the transverse nasal crease, which is a result of a child with allergies, chronically rubbing their nose.

The regular menstrual cycles and the fact that she is not taking oral contraceptive pills rules out hormonal rhinitis. Oh yeah, in this case if the question states she is not sexually active then she is not sexually active and does not have pregnancy induced hormonal rhinitis.

The patient is afebrile and therefore, is not likely to have an upper respiratory tract infection caused by rhinovirus. Rhinitis medicamentosa is associated with the use of nasal sprays containing oxymetazoline. This patient was not taking any medications.

The absence of eosinophils on nasal smear rules out non-allergic rhinitis with eosinophils or NARES.

Answers

306) **E)** The girl in this vignette self-treated herself with an over the counter medication that initially helped her. However, after a 3-4 day hiatus her nasal congestion got much worse. If her friend were a medical doctor, she would have been told not to use this medication for more than 3-4 days since it will result in rebound congestion.

She most likely took an over the counter medication containing **oxymetazoline**, which is the active ingredient in Afrin® and similar generic knock-offs. Congestion associated with **oxymetazoline** overuse is called **rhinitis medicamentosa**. The beefy, red turbinates is further evidence that this is the correct answer

The regular menstrual cycles and the fact that she is not taking oral contraceptive pills rules out hormonal rhinitis. Once again, in this case if the question states she is not sexually active then she is not sexually active and does not have pregnancy induced hormonal rhinitis.

The patient is afebrile and therefore, not likely to have an upper respiratory tract infection caused by rhinovirus. The absence of eosinophils on nasal smear rules out non-allergic rhinitis with eosinophils or NARES.

307) **B)** With a diagnosis of rhinitis medicamentosa, nasal oxymetazoline was the cause of the problem. Therefore, it cannot be the problem and the solution. Oral oxymetazoline is just a curveball we threw in for good measure , which might have led you to believe that you needed to choose between oral and nasal oxymetazoline.

Appropriate treatment would include nasal corticosteroids, while weaning off the oxymetazoline.

308) **D)** Appropriate treatment for rhinitis medicamentosa could include nasal irrigation, nasal corticosteroids, nasal antihistamines, such as azelastine and nasal mast cell stabilizers such as olopatadine.

Oxymetazoline is an intranasal medication, which could lead to rhinitis medicamentosa if used longer than 3 days. Oxymetazoline is what caused the rhinitis medicamentosa in the first place. Therefore, of all the choices listed it would be the most inappropriate choice.

309) D) Non-allergic rhinitis with eosinophils is similar to allergic rhinitis. It can be due to many triggers including hair spray and chlorine, which the girl in the vignette has been exposed to. In addition, the absence of itchy eyes points away from allergic rhinitis. The absence of discolored turbinates is additional history that points away from an allergic cause.

The regular menstrual cycles and the fact that she is not taking oral contraceptive pills rules out hormonal rhinitis. Once again if the question notes that she is not sexually active then she is not sexually active and does not have pregnancy induced hormonal rhinitis.

The patient is afebrile and therefore, not likely to have an upper respiratory tract infection caused by rhinovirus. Rhinitis medicamentosa is associated with the use of nasal sprays containing oxymetazoline. This patient was not taking any medications.

Answers

Adolescent Medicine and Gynecology

310) C) Breast development consisting of glandular tissue beyond the areolae with no secondary mounding of the nipples or areolae is a description of a sexual maturity rating of 3 for breast development.

311) D) The history is most consistent with non-specific vaginitis. Eighty percent of prepubertal vaginitis results in negative bacterial and fungal cultures. Referral to child protective services in this case would not be appropriate. Reassurance that the discharge is normal is the most appropriate management.

312) D) The HCT has dropped, there were no symptoms prior to the injury, and all other blood tests are normal. Therefore the most likely diagnosis is a deep tissue hematoma and the fatigue is due to the relative anemia.

Osteogenic sarcoma often presents in active adolescents and is first diagnosed incidentally when pain persists after an injury and is out of proportion to the level of trauma incurred. The initial symptoms are often mistakenly attributed to pain secondary to the injury. However, this child exhibits none of the other signs of osteogenic sarcoma and has all normal blood tests.

Osteoid osteoma usually presents as recurrent acute intense sudden pain at night and at rest relieved by ibuprofen, and there is nothing in the history to suggest this as the cause of the pain.

313) E) Pour a tub of Gatorade® over them and ask "Cool enough for you guys?" Providing unrestricted access to fluids is the best way to prevent heat-related illnesses. Solar generated fans as of publication date are not FDA approved.

314) C) The question clearly states that the reason for the symptoms is a recurrent chlamydia urethritis so gonococcal urethritis would not be the explanation. Azithromycin should be adequate treatment so a broader spectrum antibiotic isn't necessary. There is nothing to suggest poor compliance with one treatment. However nothing is stated regarding his partner being treated as well, therefore the most likely explanation is reinfection by his untreated partner who is there now and can be evaluated and treated as well.

315) C) A quick albeit not exact estimate of ideal body weight for females is 100 pounds for 60 inches in height plus 5 pounds for each additional inch.

For males the formula is 106 pounds for 60 inches plus 6 pounds for each additional inch.

316) A) Severe bradycardia, hypotension, hypothermia, and arrhythmias are all indications for hospital admission in a patient with anorexia nervosa. Tachycardia in an otherwise stable patient would not be an indication for hospital admission.

317) C) The patient in this vignette is experiencing moderate dysfunctional uterine bleeding. Moderate bleeding consists of cycles lasting less than 3 weeks or menses lasting more than 7 days with a hemoglobin greater than 10.

Treatment of moderate dysfunctional uterine bleeding consists of oral contraceptive pills and close follow up including serial hematocrits. Iron supplements and maintenance of a menstrual calendar would be appropriate in any adolescent female even those not experiencing dysfunctional uterine bleeding.

A packed red cell transfusion would not be indicated in any clinically stable patient.

Answers

318) D) Nuclear acid amplification testing of *patient* obtained vaginal swab sample would be the preferred method of routine sampling. If the question asked about legal documentation then a culture would be appropriate.

If the choice for nuclear acid amplification testing came down to doctor or patient provided vaginal swab sampling the answer would be patient obtained since it is just as reliable and less invasive.

Nuclear acid amplification testing is better than nuclear hybridization testing of urine.

319) B) Yes, in the states that allow it, you are expected to provide a prescription for all sexual partners within the past **60 days**, even without an evaluation. This is called expedited partner therapy (EPT).[20]

320) C) Energy drinks do contain guarana. However, it does not offset the cardiovascular effects of caffeine. Hypertension is among the cardiac risks of concern. In fact, guarana contains guaranine which is considered to be more potent than caffeine with a more prolonged effect. It's safety, effectiveness and purity is not even known at this time. As a result we can assume it is basically worse than caffeine.

There is *no* recommended minimal daily allowance of caffeine, just a recommendation not to exceed more than 300 mg daily. The caffeine content of energy drinks isn't even measured by the FDA as they do for cola drinks so it is hard to determine how much caffeine in some of them.

Because of its diuretic effects, energy drinks containing caffeine increase rather than decrease the risk for dehydration in athletes.

Ginseng is a common ingredient in energy drinks and is linked to breast tenderness and amenorrhea. Of course that is also a sign of pregnancy, therefore after you have obtained a negative Beta HCG test, rule out energy drink.

321) E) Caffeine withdrawal and/or caffeine use in excess of 300 mg of caffeine a day can result in both insomnia and drowsiness depending on whether the person is withdrawing or drank coffee or an energy drink late in the day. Osteoporosis is a health risk associated with long-term caffeine intake. Irritability is another common short-term effect. Urinary *frequency* rather than urinary incontinence is another short-term effect of caffeine since it is a diuretic.

---

20 Centers for Disease Control and Prevention. *Legal Status of Expedited Partner Treatment—Summary Totals.* Accessed November 20, 2012 at http://www.cdc.gov/std/ept/legal/totals.htm.

Sports Medicine

322) D) Well controlled seizure would not preclude participation in power lifting competition, neither would ADHD requiring stimulant medication.

Post exertional syncope is a common finding and considered to be benign. By the way it is to be distinguished from exercise associated collapse which occurs during exertion. This correlates with long QT syndrome which warrants a cardiology workup. Children with blood pressure greater than 95th percentile for age warrant additional evaluation but greater than 99% would preclude participation in power lifting.

323) D) Male teens should have at least 7-10% body fat, therefore 10% would be appropriate not high. A body fat content of 14-17% is considered to be low in young female athletes, therefore 15% would not be considered high. Long distance runners, and in fact all athletes, needing to lose weight should do so gradually under medical supervision, monitoring caloric intake closely.

Cyclic weight loss is never good, and is in fact a warning sign of binge eating and a possible eating disorder.

324) D) Proper form can be practiced with **little or no weights**, rather than with heavy weights, in anticipation of lifting heavier weights later on, so even prepubertal children can participate in these programs. Most injuries are indeed due to mishandling of weights, rather than from the actual lifting of the weights. Supervision is critical to ensure proper technique and prevent injury. Hypertension greater than 99th percentile precludes weight training therefore documentation of normotension is crucial.

Well-designed resistance training programs *can be* safe and beneficial in athletes as young as 6.

Answers

325) D) Children are indeed more likely to engage in organized sports when parents are supportive. This should not come as a surprise, since beyond emotional support and permission slips, organized sports often require money and transportation. .

A child who is physically active is more likely to be physically active in adulthood. However, there is no known correlation with lowered risk for coronary heart disease. At least nothing proven as of this writing. Lower socioeconomic status correlates with lower rates of participation in sports. Only 1/3, not 2/3, of high school students meet the CDC recommendation for 60 minutes of moderate to vigorous physical activity daily.

326) C) Medial collateral ligament strain is a very common football injury. There is rarely swelling or effusion; an effusion would instead suggest an intraarticular injury such as an anterior cruciate ligament tear. In addition, with an anterior cruciate (ACL) tear, there is often a history of a popping or snapping at the time of injury.

A lateral collateral ligament strain would present with lateral knee pain made worse with varus stress applied on examination. **Medial** collateral ligament pain is associated with pain with **valgus** stress. **Lateral** collateral ligament pain is associated with **varus** stress. Our noting that he can walk up and down stairs without locking points away from a meniscus tear.

Substance Abuse

327) **D)** **Phentolamine** and **nifedipine** are often used to manage hypertension in an acute overdose of amphetamine and/or methamphetamine. The N-methyl group actually results in an **increase** of the peripheral side effects. The D-form is 5 times more effective than the L-form. Neuroleptics are sometimes used for acute agitation and delirium.

However, Haldol's onset of action is too slow to have practical application in acute situations, and other forms such as **droperidol** are used. Amphetamines primary mechanism of action is the increased release of intracellular stores of catecholamines.

328) **B)** The most likely explanation in this clinical setting would be glue inhalation. This would not necessarily be deliberate but a distinct possibility in a camp setting. For example this could result if there were an arts and crafts activity using glue containing toluene in a poorly ventilated room.

The key to picking the correct answer is how quickly the symptoms wear off once the child is in the open air.

329) **B)** The most likely cause of sudden death due to cocaine toxicity would be a cardiac arrhythmia.

330) **A)** Alprazolam is a benzodiazepine. This could account for the sluggish presentation as well as the equal pupils which are reacting slowly. Marijuana abuse could present similarly but noting the lack of conjunctival injection is the hint that this is not the correct diagnosis.

With heroin abuse you would expect to see constricted pupils.

Amphetamine and phencyclidine (PCP) abuse you would expect to see a more agitated if not paranoid presentation.

Answers

331) B) There is no evidence of substance abuse. However there is evidence of hyperpyrexia. Cooling the patient off is critical to reduce the risk of end organ damage. However you want to cool the temperature down to 101.8 but no lower.

Providing a cool glass of water to a patient with blunted mental status would be inappropriate.

332) B) Although electronic cigarettes are used by adults for smoking cessation, there is *no evidence* that this is effective. The key to smoking cessation is counseling and if medication were to be used *bupropion* would be the medication of choice. The vapor exhaled by users may indeed contain nicotine. In addition, the vaporization technique and nicotine content are not closely regulated by the FDA at this time. These devices often are flavored making them attractive to children and certainly to teenagers. Unlike cigarettes there is no advertising limitations in place. There is no current FDA ban on flavoring of e-cigarettes.

Disorders of Cognition, Language and Learning

333) B) Remember age 2 (2/4 = 50 % intelligible), age 3 (3/4 = 75% intelligible), age 4 (4/4 = 100% intelligible). You might be tempted to choose D, but you probably haven't had a lengthy conversation with an 18 year old lately.

334) B) Since observers are biased and observation at one point in time (office visit) is unreliable, provider examination alone, and asking parents their opinion of their child's development alone is not sufficient to assess development. The only way to assess development is to use a standardized developmental screen at every well child visit. Even though monitoring vision and hearing is important, a child with normal vision and hearing can still have developmental delays.

335) E) This is a classic description of fragile X syndrome and DNA testing is much more sensitive than karyotype to order to rule it out (or in).

Answers

Behavior and Mental Health

336) C) Topiramate and imipramine have been show to help reduce binge eating. Serotonin reuptake inhibitors such as sertraline and citalopram have been shown to be helpful as well. Lisdexamfetamine has recently been approved for treatment of binge eating but only in those 18 years of age or older. The patient in this vignette was noted to be 16 years of age. Once again reading the details of the question including taking note of the age of the patient is important.

337) D) It would be prudent to at least rule out thyroid or other medical conditions that could explain the clinical picture. In addition it is important to assess the risk for suicide in any patient who is depressed. Interviewing the patient and parents separately would help identify any recent situational factors that could be triggering or contributing to the apparent depressive symptoms.

The boy in the vignette is demonstrating serious signs of clinical depression and just counseling and providing followup in 3 months would not be appropriate. He needs intervention and much closer supervision.

338) D) Learning disabilities are common in children with ADHD and **may** manifest after 3rd grade, especially when the ADHD component has been managed with medications. Since the problems seems to be occurring exclusively at school and when he has to do homework, it suggests that learning, and not behavior per se, is the issue.

Children with learning difficulties often act out when they are frustrated and unable to learn properly. Therefore in this situation the most appropriate next step would be to obtain a psychoeducational evaluation to identify any specific learning disability. Once identified, appropriate modifications can be implemented. Hopefully with such modifications in place the child's sense of frustration will diminish and along with it the acting out behaviors.

339) D) Children who are exhibiting oppositional defiant behavior whether or not they carry that diagnosis are challenging to care for. Parents must learn ways to manage the behavior in a constructive way while setting limits. This is easier said than done. Some kids within the same family are just easier to manage than others. It must be done within the context of the family; one cannot expect the child to be introspective and modify their own behavior. Medications might or might not be indicated, but Lisdexamfetamine is primarily indicated for attention deficit and not opposition-defiance and is not the first step. Therefore choice E is incorrect

Pointing out that the behavior of other children is better isn't going to work. A behavioral management modification program would be the most appropriate first step in modifying the behavior in a productive fashion that will lead to the child being a well-functioning adult operating within the limits of society

340) E) Inattention and hyperactivity must be seen in at least 2 settings to help establish the diagnosis. Typically they are observed both at home and at school, preferably by more than one teacher. Response to stimulant medication is not considered an appropriate diagnostic method.

Learning disabilities are often seen in children with ADHD, whether or not they are treated successfully for ADHD with stimulant medication. In fact, once the noise of the ADHD symptoms are quieted down, the learning disability often becomes more apparent, much like you can't see the stars while the sun is shining. Early cognitive milestones are often normal in children with ADHD. In fact abnormal cognitive milestones, if presented in the question, would likely suggest another diagnosis, and that should be your clue.

Answers

Psychosocial

341) C) Of all the risk factors listed, teens dealing with sexual identity issues, including homosexuality, are at the highest risk for suicide.

342) D) The delay of developmental milestones is the main sign of intellectual disability, formerly known as mental retardation. However, marked delays in psychomotor skills in the first year of life is more a feature of more **severe** intellectual disability.

Normal motor development with delayed speech and language abilities in the toddler years is more typical of **moderate** intellectual disability.

On the other hand, **mild** intellectual disability is usually not suspected until after entry into school. Participation in an organized preschool can highlight discrepancies prior to school entry, but they are *most likely* to be diagnosed at school entry.

343) A) Autism has not been associated with trisomy 21. However, all of the other choices listed are associated with autism. Other conditions not listed, which include neurofibromatosis, encephalitis, maternal rubella, and infantile spasms are associated with autism.

344) C) Dyslexia is the *most common* developmental language disorder. It is frequently diagnosed in the 4th grade, when a child is called upon to use the reading skills learned in earlier grades. However, children with high cognitive abilities can sometimes compensate. If there is adequate compensation, then the diagnosis often doesn't occur until adulthood, if at all. Autopsies of adults with dyslexia have resulted in the documentation of a possible anatomical basis for the disease.

345) C) A 3-year-old with an otherwise normal history and physical exam who has marked speech delay should be assumed to have a hearing deficit until proven otherwise. Appropriate identification and intervention should be a top priority.

The following table is a rough guideline of red flags by age to keep in mind to determine when a hearing evaluation would be indicated. This is important when presented with a similar history on the exam, and should help you decide when a hearing screen would be the appropriate answer:

Age	Deficit
1 year old	Lack of vocal imitation
1-1/2 year old	The inability to use single words
2 year old	A vocabulary of less than 10 words
3 year old (the patient in the vignette)	A vocabulary of less than 200 words and less than 1/2 their words are understood

346) B) An infant who is older than 6 months but younger than 9 months should be able to babble and transfer an object from one hand to the other. A child less than 9 months old wouldn't be able to hold two objects; likewise they would not be able to lift their bellies off the floor until age 9 months.

Most 18-year-olds can and will babble and transfer a cube from one hand to another; however, one of the objects would have to be an I-Pod®.

347) B) These milestones are most consistent with that of a 2-month-old infant. A child of 2 months should be able to lift his head while lying down. An infant will be able to hold a rattle at 4 months.

348) D) Adopted children should be informed when their verbal skills and comprehension are adequate to grasp the information. The topic should be brought up naturally when appropriate, i.e., at the birth of other relatives or friends or when reading a story. The topic should be discussed when the child wishes to, and information appropriate to age and developmental stage should be available. However, it should not be discussed in excess. Discussing the subject when it naturally comes up would be the best way to "normalize" the situation.

Answers

349) E) There is no evidence that any herbal or supplemental medications work in the treatment of ADHD. Likewise there is also no evidence that dyes, preservatives, or sugar in the diet cause or worsens this condition. A multimodal approach including stimulant[21] medication and behavioral interventions is the most successful approach to managing ADHD. Often the results are dramatic; around 70% of kids respond favorably to stimulant medication.

350) A) This is one of those questions on approach and ethics. Clearly the first choice is the only one that would not alienate the parents and would get them to agree to this important procedure. However surgery cannot wait another 6 months.

351) C) The combination of "ritualistic", "withdrawn" behavior coupled with tantrums at 24 months of age is typical for autism. Autism is also characterized by abnormal language development. Stranger anxiety would not be an issue since autistic children show lack of closeness to the parents. They would not necessarily distinguish parent from stranger.

352) E) Although some 18-month-olds might know more than 12 words, the use of considerable jargon is normal for a child that age.[22] The use of 2-word sentences would also not be "normal" at this stage; it is a 24-month skill. Therefore, reassurance is the correct answer as is often the case on the exam and in practice.

353) D) **Sexual orientation** is refers to the physical and emotional arousal toward other people. Is the gender, male or female, that a person identifies with?

Sexual orientation is biologically based but is determined by genetic, hormonal and environmental influences

Homosexual teens are at a *higher risk* to drop out than their heterosexual peers.

Sexual orientation is *not a choice* and therefore parents should not be told that their children are *free to choose* their sexual orientation.

However sexual behavior and activity are choices teens make.

---

[21] And, when contraindicated, other medications.
[22] As well as pediatricians at major meetings.

354) D) Vaginal discharge and irritation could be due to physiologic vaginitis. Interest in wearing men's clothing would not be abnormal and neither would reluctance to undress in front of the mother.

However imitation of adult sexual activities would not be expected or normal and would warrant further investigation.

355) B) A child with a progressively debilitating illness will be aware of the severity of their condition. The most appropriate option would be to explain to the child consistent with their developmental ability to understand.

356) B) Peak onset of separation anxiety disorder is middle childhood around age 7-9 the symptoms can persist into early adulthood, including difficulty with going away to college.

Children with separation anxiety disorder often have other psychiatric disorders.

Some studies show that it occurs primarily in females, but new studies show increasing prevalence among males.

357) D) It is recommended that children resume regular school attendance without the parent present and without gradual withdrawal of parents.

This might seem to contradict the exposure based cognitive behavioral therapy which emphasizes gradual introduction of fearful situations. However this stage is best done cold turkey because a child's anxiety tends to decrease soon after a parent leaves.

Answers

Critical Care

358) C) The formula is 7 ml/kg and therefore 100ml is the closest. I believe 6 trillion would be the correct answer if you were asked to calculate the number of people who voted more than once on American Idol, but this is of course beyond the scope of this book.

359) D) Botulism toxin acts by blocking the release of acetylcholine from the presynaptic neuron.

360) D) Prompt CPR including mouth to mouth resuscitation coupled with chest compressions can prove to be life saving and is the most important step to take immediately after a child is rescued from a near drowning episode.

Attempts to clear the airway including the Heimlich maneuver are not helpful and may prove to be more harmful by inducing emesis instead.

361) B) Noncardiogenic pulmonary edema, impaired oxygenation, and bilateral pulmonary infiltrates is the diagnostic triad of ARDS. However the clinical manifestations can consist of tachypnea, diminished lung compliance, and increasing hypoxemia which ultimately result in respiratory failure secondary to muscle fatigue.

ARDS usually occurs soon after lung injury secondary to drowning, however it can occur hours and even days after initial lung injury.

ARDS is due to *alveolar capillary insult resulting in increased pulmonary capillary permeability.*

In addition to drowning RDS can be secondary to:

- Pneumonia
- Aspiration
- Lung contusion
- Smoke inhalation
- Blood product transfusion
- Sepsis

Emergency Medicine

362) C) Sodium bicarbonate cannot be administered via an ET tube. You can use the mnemonic LANE to help remember that **lidocaine, atropine, naloxone HCl and epinephrine** can all be administered via an endotracheal tube.

363) B) The clinical picture is the deciding factor in determining whether to discharge a child with bronchiolitis rather than the etiology. The use of racemic epinephrine could result in resumption of symptoms after initial improvement as a rebound effect. Therefore, a period of observation and/or admission would be appropriate.

364) B) An abuse pattern will more typically appear with different degrees of variation in shade and not be uniform in color (such as are Mongolian spots and the discoloration they are describing). The strawberry hemangiomas will typically become worse prior to involuting. No intervention is needed unless it is large enough and in an area that could potentially interfere with function, for example, near the eyelid where it would obstruct vision.

365) C) Except for beta blockers all of the other choices can be indicated under certain conditions and be safely used to manage acute methamphetamine intoxications.

Beta-blockers alone should not be used because the unopposed alpha stimulation can be life threatening.

If reduction of blood pressure is the goal, an **alpha-blocker** such as **phentolamine** and a **vasodilator** such as **nifedipine** would be better choices.

Seizures can be controlled with benzodiazepines such as lorazepam.

Answers

366) **E)** This child is exhibiting *Cushing's triad*, which is seen in patients with increased intracranial pressure and consists of:

1. Hypertension
2. Bradycardia
3. Irregular respirations

A lumbar puncture would not only be unhelpful but also contraindicated in the face of increased intracranial pressure. None of the other steps would address the main problem except for *hyperventilation*, which induces hypocarbia, resulting in cerebral vasoconstriction and decreased cerebral blood flow.

367) **A)** The clinical scenario is that of *opiate overdose*. Administering naloxone would initially be diagnostic (pupil dilating) and ultimately therapeutic as more is given once diagnosis is confirmed

Clearly glucose would be contraindicated in a patient who is already hyperglycemic.

368) **C)** Cardiac arrhythmias such as inverted T-waves and depressed ST segments would be the most "serious" consequences of glue sniffing. Management in the acute situation is directed toward monitoring for cardiac arrhythmias above all else.

369) **E)** Since this child is on chronic systemic steroids, adrenal suppression is very likely. Therefore, administering perioperative steroids IV would be indicated.

370) **C)** Administration of insulin and glucose would actually be an appropriate method to treat hyperkalemia. Cardiorespiratory monitoring would certainly be appropriate and necessary to monitor for any cardiac arrhythmias that might develop as a result.

371) D) Although the typical presentation of pyelonephritis might be "flank pain" or CVA[23] tenderness, **pyelonephritis can also present as RUQ tenderness**. The pain, chills, and vomiting suggest infection of the upper urinary tract and not just "cystitis".

There is nothing in this vignette to suggest renal stones. The positive urine culture makes cholecystitis and gallstones unlikely.

372) D) Despite the relatively benign physical examination including a GCS of 14, the history of loss of consciousness coupled with the vomiting would warrant a CT scan. Overnight observation would be indicated as well, but the head CT would not be dependent on observed clinical status during the hospital stay, it would precede the admission.

373) A) This is a classic description of PCP (phencyclidine) ingestion. Hyperreflexia is associated with PCP ingestion.

With higher levels of PCP ingestion, patients can become comatose and hypotensive. *However, respiratory depression is rare and more consistent with opiate overdose.*

374) E) This is a *septal hematoma* and essentially a surgical emergency. If the hematoma is not evacuated and proper surgical intervention implemented, it will result in compromised blood supply to the cartilage and a *"saddle nose" deformity*. This is the typical deformity seen in old boxers and extras on the set of all of the "Rocky" movies.

375) C) Once again, rarely is something mentioned without a reason. The child has an unremarkable history and comes to the ER lethargic. **Noting that the mother is being treated for depression is important and suggestive of a toxic ingestion.**

Syrup of ipecac is no longer recommended for anything, anytime, anywhere.

The most likely ingested medication is a tricyclic antidepressant which is a board favorite. Tricyclic ingestion can result in cardiac arrhythmias, making the EKG an appropriate step. Although not listed, alkalinization of the urine would also be appropriate.

Certainly, protecting the airway of a lethargic child could never be an incorrect choice. Once intubated, administration of charcoal via an NG tube could be indicated.

---

[23] Costovertebral angle.

Answers

376) E) Answer E would be consistent with Caffey disease, which also goes by the name *infantile cortical hyperostosis*. A metaphyseal fracture,[24] also known as a "bucket handle" fracture, is virtually always secondary to abuse. While a child who is ice-skating may fall a lot, rib fractures are very unlikely to be "accidental" unless they were playing hockey against teenagers (the same would apply to a skull fracture). Although bruising of the shins is very common in 2-year-olds you would not expect to see evidence of "multiple fractures" unless there was a result of a non accidental injury.

377) A) Deferoxamine binds free iron in the serum and forms ferrioxamine, a water soluble, renally excreted compound which, if present, turns the urine a characteristic reddish-orange or "vin rose" color.

378) E) Neglect is the most common form of child abuse.

379) C) Any child exhibiting vomiting and lethargy following a head injury requires prompt evaluation. Skull films have no place; it is either Head CT or no studies.

380) C) Ketamine has the potential to *increase* not decrease secretions. Therefore, it is often used with atropine to counter this effect. It works primarily via sensory blockade and is often used for short painful procedures.

One of the problems with ketamine is it can produce a dreamlike state, with hallucinations *before* the sensory blockade takes effect. The last thing you want is a patient hallucinating in anticipation of a painful procedure. That is why midazolam is often used together with ketamine.

---

24 Not to be confused with a metaphysical fracture, which is a fracture from reality!

381) A) Midazolam's usefulness in conscious sedation is due to its amnesic, anxiolytic, and sedative effects. It has no *analgesic effect.*

I would say that anything which an anxiolytic, amnesic and sedating is quite enigmatic. The important point to remember is that midazolam has no analgesic benefits and if a procedure is painful, another agent must be used as well.

382) D) The most likely diagnosis would be intussusception. Intussusception presents between ages 3 months – 3 years, with intermittent episodes of vomiting with lethargy in between episodes in a child who is afebrile. In addition to the classic currant jelly stools, bilious vomiting could also be part of the presenting picture. On x-ray, specifically air or contrast enema can reveal the lead point as a "coiled spring" appearance.

If you see the words coiled spring in the description and intussusception as one of the answers, you can for all intents and purposes break out the cork screw to open the champagne en route to your taking another step toward passing the exam.

383) D) The patient is presenting with classic signs of scarlet fever and strep pharyngitis. The rash is the classic sandpaper rash. Strep can often present with sore throat, of course, headache, rash and abdominal pain severe enough to mimic acute appendicitis. Therefore the most appropriate next step would be rapid strep and throat culture

384) E) The most likely explanation for the presentation would be new onset diabetic ketoacidosis (DKA) which can often present as acute abdominal pain. In this case the other signs including weight loss, weakness and polyuria as well as polydipsia are other classic signs of diabetes type 1.

The acetone odor is consistent with ketones not glue sniffing. In this case perhaps it is the coach who is sniffing glue not seeing these classic signs.

Answers

Pharmacology and Pain Management

385) E) St. John's wort can decrease the efficacy of oral contraceptive pills by inducing the cytochrome P-450 pathway speeding up the elimination of oral contraceptive pills and decreasing its bioavailability.

386) A) Echinacea is contraindicated in patients taking immunosuppressant medications. Just note this; it will come in handy on the exam.

387) B) Ginseng can interact with oral hypoglycemic agents, oral anticoagulants, antiplatelet agents as well as corticosteroids.

388) B) The fact that it is BID is not really relevant. What is relevant is that a steady state (no not Maryland) is achieved in 5 days (5 twenty-four hour periods) and that it takes 5 half lives to reach a steady state. Therefore, the half-life is closest to one day, which is 24 hours.

389) D) Hypertension does not alter the serum levels of medications. All of the other choices have the potential to alter serum albumin levels, and anything that alters serum albumin alters the effectiveness of a variety of medications. Juvenile polyps reduce the serum albumin level because of general protein loss.

Research and Statistics

390) D) A Cohort study ranks second only to Randomized Controlled Trials with respect to Internal Validity. A cohort study investigates the causes of disease by establishing links between risk factors and health outcomes. .

A "cohort", or sample of individuals with and without a risk factor, are followed over time either forward for a future outcome (prospective), or traced backward for a historic risk (retrospective) to see if they develop a health outcome. Clearly, time sequence is one of the benefits of cohort studies.

Strengths of Cohort studies are that they establish the risk of a particular exposure (does going out with wet hair really cause pneumonia?) and that they are inexpensive to do retrospectively (how many of those pneumonia kids had not listened to their mother and gone out with wet hair?).

A weakness of cohort studies is that they require a large sample size so it's difficult to study rare outcomes. (Does going out with wet hair cause *Legionella* pneumonia?). Also, since prospective cohort studies take place over time, you often lose subjects to follow up. , Prospective cohort studies can get expensive and it is difficult to control for confounding variables (was it also winter, or did they already have the sniffles when they went out with the wet hair?).

391) E) Most busy pediatricians do not have the time or resource to parse through studies and must rely on review articles.

Those who choose to write review articles, of course, must know how to determine which studies are valid and which are not. This is where understanding the process of systematic review and meta-analysis comes in. Even if you don't plan on ever writing a review article, questions on the subject are fair game, and answering them correctly could be the difference between passing and failing the boards.

What is systematic review? It's exactly what it says. A systematic review is a complete review of the literature on a given clinical question or topic. But it is not so simple, otherwise there could be no board questions on the subject. There is a uniform specific method you must adhere to when "searching and reviewing the literature"

Therefore, choice B is incorrect. The search is not *random*. There is a rigorous specific protocol.

All published studies do not have to be included in the review. However, the article must explain the criteria for study inclusion and exclusion in the review. For example, the review may only choose to include studies involving patients under age 12, or only asthmatics who are on daily corticosteroids, or children with only one specific seizure type.

Answers

Publication bias is a result of authors more likely submitting studies with results that confirm their hypotheses than studies with findings that prove the null hypothesis. Therefore literature searches are less likely to turn up unpublished studies with **negative findings**. One way to correct this bias is for journals to require pre-registration before implementing a study. This will allow literature reviews to include unpublished studies that prove the null hypothesis without being null and void regarding the literature search.

So what's the matter with meta-analysis and what the heck is it? A meta-analysis pools all the data from multiple related studies and draws one statistical conclusion.

Meta-analysis is an additional step but **not necessarily a part of an adequate systematic literature review**. For example, it is not needed if the existing research is too limited or the research done is too different for the meta-analysis to be relevant.

The Cochrane library *is* an independent compilation of systematic reviews of medical topics. Therefore, choice E is correct

392) C) Meta-analysis pools all the data from multiple related studies and draws one statistical conclusion. Studies that include more subjects get more weight. Therefore, the summary of pooled statistics are weighted to favor larger studies.

Homogeneity and heterogeneity have nothing to do with political correctness. Homogeneity refers to studies that were conducted similarly. For example, if the data was collected by subjective self-examination vs ultrasound.

Studies that have data from patients are like comparing apples to apples. As a result, these studies have a higher homogeneity. Studies that have, for example, data that is self-reported and data from objective imaging data, the studies have a higher heterogeneity are more like comparing apples to oranges. **Homogeneity and heterogeneity are important factors in the meta-analysis of pooled studies.**

Studies that demonstrate negative results that are statistically relevant are less likely to get published. If at all possible these should be included in the meta-analysis since their absence results in publication bias.

393) C) A case control study, as the name implies, looks at two groups. Those 2 groups are the "case" and "study" groups. The case group has a disease or something of interest. The control group does not have this disease of thing of interest. In conducting the study, one looks back through the retroscope to look for the exposure of a risk factor for both groups.

Since you are studying a group that already has a given exposure of condition, it is an excellent way to study rare disease with long latency periods. Since the groups are already set up, it is *not* very time consuming. Since you already have one group with a condition and one without it, is *not* a good method to study diagnostic tests.

One of the advantages of the case control study is you *can* study *multiple* risk factors.

394) B) In a randomized controlled study, there is an experimental group and a control group. It is best done in a double blind setting, where the groups and those conducting the study are unaware of who is in each group. The results can then be analyzed with established statistical tools. However setting up and running such studies does not come cheap.

If participants are volunteers, it blunts the randomization, which is an important component of the study. Therefore, volunteer participation presents a "volunteer bias"

Ideally the only variation between the control and the experimental group is the variable being studied. Additional "confounding" variables can diminish the validity of the findings.

And even if you manage to control the variables, a randomized controlled trial study can demonstrate correlation, but it does not necessarily demonstrate causation.

Ethics for Primary Care Physicians

395) D) While counseling and multispecialty evaluation is certainly indicated in the treatment of transgender youth, management prior to adulthood is not limited to this., Long term outcome is best if pubertal suppression, hormonal therapy, and gender reassignment surgery are all performed prior to adulthood.

Although not FDA approved, pubertal suppression through gonadotropin-releasing hormone (GnRH) analogs does allow for a smoother social and physical transition to the gender role congruent with gender identity. The child must be peri-pubertal. This would be considered inappropriate in a pre-pubertal child since gender non-conforming behaviors are common and not necessarily an indication of evolving transgender identity.

Psychiatric comorbidity is very common among transgender youth, including depression, anxiety and high risk for suicide. The pediatrician is expected to be on the lookout for signs of gender dysphoria, couched in general signs of depression , school failure, and other signs of psychological distress. Therefore choice E is incorrect.

Adolescents are unlikely to broach the subject of GD with their physicians, and parents often have not identified the problem to that degree of specificity. Accordingly, the primary care clinician must have a high index of suspicion and persist in gathering pertinent history.

396) E) When it comes to living solid organ donation by a sibling several criteria must be met. In addition to parental consent, the minor child must "assent" to the decision. The lower age range for mandatory assent is 11-14 years of age. Therefore choice B and C are not correct. In general, avoid choices that state "never" and "always".

Regarding solid organ donation, this assent must be established by an independent advocacy board to avoid conflict of interest. Parents conceiving with the hopes have having a child who is a good match, serving as a savior sibling, is considered ethical provided that child is cared for and loved in his or her own right.

397) E) Regarding implementation of of bioelectromagnetic or any alternative treatment options, several factors must be considered.

ND the wishes of the parents should be considered. However, it is important to review any potential adverse effects and it should be used with, rather than instead of, traditional evidence based management.

398) D) While vaccines are very effective with a favorable risk/ benefit ratio, it would be inappropriate to assure parents that any vaccine is 100% safe or effective. Regarding the general community, parents who refuse to immunize *their* children are benefitting from the risk other families take by immunizing their children. The lower prevalence of disease in the community results in herd immunity. The more pejorative term for this situation is "free riders". Not only are these parents benefitting from the risk taken by other families who participate in recommended vaccine programs, they are also increasing the risk for other members of the community. Specifically, even in a fully immunized population, there are children with conditions that place them at increased risk for disease. Should the unimmunized child contract the preventable disease, they are placing these vulnerable children at increased risk despite *their* parents taking all the steps to reduce their child's risk. It becomes a question of justice and public health.

Regarding measles disease and vaccine, the risk for encephalopathy with the vaccine is 1 / 1 million. The risk for encephalopathy for those who contract measles is 1 / 1 thousand.

399) A) It is perfectly acceptable to have expert testimony submitted to a panel of peers for review. In other words, assume that your peers will have the opportunity to put you on the hot seat, so be careful what you say. Even in the absence of this possibility, the guidelines for testimony mandate that testimony is based on medical evidence and the standards of practice. It is considered ethical to appear in court as a witness whether mandated to do so or not. We are expected to assist in the legal process where medical issues related to our specialty is involved. Getting paid "market value" for providing services is also acceptable. But it should go without saying, the compensation cannot be contingent on the outcome. Although it might not serve you well, testifying against a colleague you have to work with is not considered to be unethical. In some cases, courts have required that the testifying doctor must be from the same state, so that the standards of practice closely match. This is called "locality rules".

Answers

Patient Safety and Quality Improvement

400) B) A sentinel event is an unanticipated event in a healthcare setting that results in death or serious physical or psychological injury or the risk thereto that occurs as a *result of medical care*. Therefore choice B is the correct answer

A sentinel event can be the result of a medical error but not all sentinel events are the result of medical error. However, a sentinel event by definition requires further investigation.

401) D) You are expected to understand and know the nuanced differences between various errors that can occur as a result of a breakdown in the implementation of medical treatment.

A medical error is defined as a "failure to complete a planned action as intended, or the use of a wrong plan to achieve an aim."

Therefore Choice D is the correct answer.

402) C) A near miss event is a medical error that places a patient at risk of injury but does not result in harm.

Near miss events can either be *intercepted* before impacting the patient or they can be *non-intercepted*.

Near miss events do not cause harm to the patient regardless of whether they are intercepted or not. For example if a child received a dose of ibuprofen that was 3 times the indicated dose it is unlikely that serious harm would result. Therefore choice C would be incorrect in stating that a non-intercepted near miss **always** results in harm to the patient.

A near miss event can be the result of an incorrect entry into an EMR. In the ibuprofen example above, someone may have entered the patient weight as 80kg instead of 8kg.

403) B) All adverse events by definition result in harm to the patient. Some are preventable, like a known penicillin-allergic patient getting penicillin, and some and non-preventable, like not having known the patient was allergic beforehand.

It is important to note that an adverse event is a result of **medical management** it is *not due to the underlying disease or condition of the patient.* Therefore all of the choices are true *except* choice B. However an adverse event is not necessarily due to medical error. An example might be an allergic reaction to amoxicillin, in a patient taking amoxicillin for the first time.

Most medical errors are not adverse events because most do not result in harm to the patient. An adverse drug event (ADE) is an adverse event that is due to medication use.

404) B) Medical errors can but do not always result in harm to the patient. **Even when there is no harm to the individual patient the error should be reviewed and tracked to determine the root cause of the error.**

A sentinel event is "an unexpected occurrence involving death or serious physical or psychological injury or the risk thereof". Although it may not lead to actual harm, it is still a close call "near miss" and is considered a golden opportunity to investigate in order to prevent this from occurring in the future. The next patient might not be so lucky.

Not all sentinel events are due to medical error. An example would be an allergic reaction to a medication that was given to a patient who had not had a reaction previously. This also means that not all adverse drug events are preventable.

References

Nutrition

1. Wagner CL, Greer FR; American Academy of Pediatrics Section on Breastfeeding; American Academy of Pediatrics Committee on Nutrition. Prevention of rickets and vitamin D deficiency in infants, children, and adolescents. Pediatrics. 2008;122(5):1142–1152

Preventive Pediatrics

2. Mercuri E, Muntoni The ever-expanding spectrum of congenital muscular dystrophies. Ann Neurol. 2012;72(1):9–17 75-78

Poisons and Toxins

3. Carvalho M, Carmo H, Costa VM, Capela JP, Pontes H, Remião F, et al. Toxicity of amphetamines: an update. *Arch Toxicol.* Mar 6 201

Infectious Disease

4. April 2009 PIR

5. Dec 2014 PRI

6. Luzuriaga K, Sullivan JL. Infectious mononucleosis. N Engl J Med. 2010;362(21): 1993–200096

Heme Onc

7. Lake AM, Oski FA. Peripheral lymphadenopathy in childhood. Ten-year experience with excisional biopsy. *Am J Dis Child.* 1978;132 :357– 359

Renal

8. Moxey-Mims M. Hematuria and proteinuria. In: Kher KK, Schnaper HW, Makker SP, eds. *Clinical Pediatric Nephrology.* 2nd ed. Abingdon, United Kingdom: Informa Healthcare; 2007:129–139.

Neurology

9. Friedman MJ, Sharieff GQ. Seizures in children. *Pediatr Clin North Am.* 2006;53:257-77.

10. Friedman MJ, Sharieff GQ. Seizures in children. *Pediatr Clin North Am.* 2006;53:257-77.

11. Friedman MJ, Sharieff GQ. Seizures in children. *Pediatr Clin North Am.* 2006;53:257-77.

Musculoskeletal

12. Bushby K, Finkel R, Birnkrant DJ, et al ; DMD Care Considerations Working Group. Diagnosis and management of Duchenne muscular dystrophy, part 1: diagnosis, and pharmacological and psychosocial management. Lancet Neurol. 2010;9(1):77–93

Ophthalmology

13. Howard GR. Eyelid retraction. In: Yanoff M, Duker JS, eds. *Ophthalmology.* 3rd ed. St. Louis, Mo: Mosby Elsevier; 2008:chap 12.4.

14. Walton KA, Buono LM. Horner syndrome. Curr Opin Ophthalmol. 2003 Dec;14(6):357-63.

ENT

15. Dykewicz, MS, Fineman, S, Skoner, DP, Nicklas, R, Lee, R et al, **Diagnosis and management of rhinitis: complete guidelines of the Joint Task Force on Practice Parameters in Allergy, Asthma, and Immunology. American Academy of Allergy, Asthma, and Immunology**. *Ann Allergy Asthma Immunol.* 1998;81:478–518

16. Wallace DV, Dykewicz MS, Bernstein DI, et al. The diagnosis and management of rhinitis: an updated practice parameter. *J Allergy Clin Immunol.* Aug 2008;122(2 Suppl):S1-84. [Medline].

17. Wallace DV, Dykewicz MS, Bernstein DI, et al. The diagnosis and management of rhinitis: an updated practice parameter. *J Allergy Clin Immunol.* Aug 2008;122(2 Suppl):S1-84. [Medline].

18. Wallace DV, Dykewicz MS, Bernstein DI, et al. The diagnosis and management of rhinitis: an updated practice parameter. *J Allergy Clin Immunol.* Aug 2008;122(2 Suppl):S1-84. [Medline].

Sports Medicine

References

19. https://2016.prepsa.courses.aap.org/course/resume-test?status=answered&cache=636101730246050360

20. https://2014.prepsa.courses.aap.org/course/resume-test?status=answered

21. http://pedsinreview.aappublications.org/content/32/5/e53#T1

22. http://www.epilepsy.com/learn/seizures-youth/about-kids/playing-sports-and-other-activities

23. https://cme.aappublications.org/events/highwire/content/p.jsp?u=aHR0cDovL2NsYXNzaWMucGVkc2lucmV2aWV3LmFhcHB1YmxpY2F0aW9ucy5vcmcvY29udGVudC8zNy8zLzExNC5mdWxsLmh0bWw_Y211LWRpc3BsYXk9dHJ1ZQ&startSpan=Radiographs%20reveal%20lytic&endSpan=sclerotic%20rim.#TSHAnchor

Behavior and Mental Health

24. https://cme.aappublications.org/events/highwire/content/p.jsp?u=aHR0cDovL2NsYXNzaWMucGVkc2lucmV2aWV3LmFhcHB1YmxpY2F0aW9ucy5vcmcvY29udGVudC84LzMyMy5mdWxsLmh0bWw_Y211LWRpc3BsYXk9dHJ1ZQ&startSpan=Accordingly%2C%20psychotherapy%2C%20particularly&endSpan=medical%20consequences%20of%20the%20disorder.#TSHAnchor

Research and Statistics

25. Porta, Miquel, ed. (2008). *A Dictionary of Epidemiology* (5th ed.). New York: Oxford University Press.

26. Kontopantelis E, Reeves D (2012). "Performance of statistical methods for meta-analysis when true study effects are non-normally distributed: A simulation study." *Statistical Methods in Medical Research* **21** (4): 409–26.

Ethics for Primary Care Physicians

27. http://pedsinreview.aappublications.org/content/37/3/89

28. http://pedsinreview.aappublications.org/content/33/2/e13

29. American Academy of Pediatrics Committee on Medical Liability. Guidelines for expert witness testimony in medical malpractice litigation. *Pediatrics*. 2002;109:974. Available at **http://pediatrics.aappublications.org/content/109/5/974.long**.

30. Jerrold L. The role of the expert witness. *Surg Clin North Am*. 2007; 87(4):889-901. DOI: **http://dx.doi.org/10.1016/j.suc.2007.07.010**.

31. The AAP recognizes that pediatricians "have the professional, ethical, and legal duty to assist in the legal process when medical issues are involved.

Patient Safety and Quality Improvements

32. 9Sentinel Events. Oakbrook Terrace, Ill: The Joint Commission; 2007. Accessed January 2010 at: http://www.jointcommission.org/SentinelEvents/

33. Woods D, Thomas E, Holl J, Altman S, Brennan T. Adverse events and preventable adverse events in children. *Pediatrics*. 2005; 115:155–160